# The Science and Engineering of Sport Surfaces

Sports surface design is crucial for the successful performance of sports skills and the reduction of injury risk. Surfaces have developed from natural materials such as turf, clay and cinder to synthetic surfaces such as acrylic tennis courts, artificial turf for soccer and synthetic running tracks, while our understanding of natural turf has developed in terms of properties appropriate for different sports and surface sustainability. This book draws together the latest research on biomechanical, medical and engineering approaches to the study of sports surfaces.

Written by a team of leading international sports scientists, engineers and technologists, the book covers every key aspect of surface development and design, including:

- surface behaviour
- surface classification, function, construction and maintenance
- influence of surfaces on player performance and injury
- surface test methods and monitoring
- development of natural turf and synthetic surfaces
- shoe–turf interaction
- future developments in sports surface technology.

Representing the most comprehensive and up-to-date study of sports surfaces, this book is important reading for all researchers and professionals working in sports technology, sports engineering, biomechanics or sports medicine.

**Sharon Dixon** is Senior Lecturer in Sports Biomechanics at the University of Exeter where she leads the Exeter Biomechanics Research Team. Her research is in improving understanding of injury mechanisms in sport and exercise, with a particular focus on footwear and playing surfaces. Her recent work has included an interdisciplinary project on natural turf surfaces with Dr Iain James and a project in collaboration with Dr Matt Carré combining biomechanical and mechanical methods to improve understanding of surfaces used in tennis and the potential influence on injury.

**Paul Fleming** is Senior Lecturer in Geotechnical Engineering at Loughborough University and leads a research team in the area of sports surface science. His background is in advanced testing of geo-materials, including a PhD in dynamic impact testing, and geotechnical design and construction experience translated into the under-researched topic sports surface science in 2001. He sits on several technical committees including the BS committee for sports surface testing (PRI/57) and he founded the global SportSURF research network in 2005.

**Iain James** is Technical Director at TGMS Ltd, a Sports Surface Design Consultancy based in the UK and delivering new construction and renovation projects from recreational to international elite sport venues. He was formerly Senior Lecturer in the School of Applied Sciences at Cranfield University in the UK, leading a research programme in Sports Surface Engineering and Technology that aimed to develop improved safety, performance and sustainability in sports surface design and construction.

**Matt Carré** is a Reader in Mechanical Engineering at the University of Sheffield and leads research in the area of human–environment interactions, including those that involve sports surfaces. His first experience of sports surfaces research was in 1996 during his PhD study that included replicating and assessing over 15,000 impacts between cricket balls and pitches. Matt has since examined traction of association football shoes and more recent work includes the development of a biomechanically informed lab-based system to simulate tennis shoe–surface interactions (in collaboration with Sharon Dixon).

## Routledge Research in Sports Technology and Engineering

The *Routledge Research in Sports Technology and Engineering* series showcases cutting-edge research from this increasingly significant discipline. Featuring the work of established and emerging scientists and practitioners from around the world, this series is an important channel for new and ground-breaking research in technology and engineering for sport.

Available in this series:

**The Science and Engineering of Sport Surfaces**
*Edited by Sharon Dixon, Paul Fleming, Iain James and Matt Carré*

# The Science and Engineering of Sport Surfaces

Edited by Sharon Dixon,
Paul Fleming, Iain James
and Matt Carré

Routledge
Taylor & Francis Group
LONDON AND NEW YORK

First published 2015
by Routledge
2 Park Square, Milton Park, Abingdon, Oxon OX14 4RN

and by Routledge
711 Third Avenue, New York, NY 10017

*Routledge is an imprint of the Taylor & Francis Group, an informa business*



*British Library Cataloguing-in-Publication Data*
A catalogue record for this book is available from the British Library

*Library of Congress Cataloging in Publication Data*
The science and engineering of sport surfaces / edited by Sharon Dixon, Paul Fleming, Iain James & Matt Carre.
pages cm
Includes bibliographical references and index.
1. Synthetic sporting surfaces. 2. Athletic fields. 3. Turf management. 4. Human mechanics. 5. Sports--Physiological aspects. I. Dixon, Sharon, editor. II. Fleming, P. (Paul), 1964- editor. III. James, Iain, editor. IV. Carre, Matt editor.
TP1185.S65S28 2015
635.9'642068--dc23
2014043133

ISBN: 978-0-415-50092-0 (hbk)
ISBN: 978-0-203-13338-5 (ebk)

Typeset in Baskerville and Gill Sans
by Saxon Graphics Ltd, Derby



MIX
Paper from responsible sources
FSC® C013056
FSC www.fsc.org

Printed and bound in Great Britain by
TJ International Ltd, Padstow, Cornwall

# Contents

# Figures

# Tables

# Foreword

*Alastair Cox*

Over the last 20 years there have been significant developments in the range of sports surfaces being used at the elite and community levels of many sports. FIFA and UEFA now allow the use of synthetic turf surfaces in all of their competitions, and hockey has moved away from playing on the traditional grass pitch to only playing on a synthetic turf surface, which no longer even has to be green in colour. Rugby, athletics, tennis, netball and a range of other sports are now all regularly played on one form of synthetic surface or another. The natural turf industry has not sat back and allowed sports to move away from the surface that many still consider to be the best playing surface. Hybrid pitches, combining natural and synthetic technologies, are now being installed in many stadia around the world, allowing increased use for sporting and non-sporting activities.

Sports governing bodies have seen the benefits of these new technologies and have encouraged their use by modifying their competition rules to allow the use of the new surfaces providing they have acceptable sports performance, player welfare and durability qualities. Measuring these properties has also seen advances in the testing methods used, but the need to develop standards relatively quickly and be able to transport the test equipment around the world often compromises the more fundamental understanding that is required to ensure new sports surfaces fully provide the playing characteristics athletes require, while also ensuring the surfaces do not have longer-term effects on health or welfare. Likewise as society generally recognises the benefits of a healthy lifestyle and of protecting the environment, the need for sports surfaces to be able to sustain much greater levels of use for longer periods of time, without having a detrimental effect on the natural world, is becoming ever more important.

While the advances in sports surface technology and testing methods are significant there is still much to be learnt and this book provides up-to-date information and research findings. It will be a useful reference for students, academics and practitioners alike with an interest in the science and practical application of sports surface science. It should greatly help advance our understanding of what constitutes a high quality, good-performing, durable yet environmentally friendly sports surface.

**Alastair Cox** is an internationally recognised expert on the performance and testing of sports surfaces. With over 35 years' experience he regularly consults with all of the major international sports governing bodies that have seen the need to assess and regulate the types of sports surface on which their sports are played.

# Preface

This book aims to provide a multidisciplinary account of the development of sports surfaces, focusing primarily on science and engineering aspects. The book has drawn on the knowledge and expertise of contributors from academia and industry, and aims to provide a useful reference to students, researchers and practitioners.

The technologies in both artificial turf and natural turf, and across a range of other indoor and outdoor surfaces, has progressed apace in the last 30 years. However there are very few books dedicated to this subject area. One book that is still relevant is that by Graham Tipp and Vic Watson, published in 1982, wherein they provided a broad but well-detailed text with useful descriptions of the emerging polymer technologies involved. Around the same time, the development of a scientific interest in sports surfaces led to a symposium on sports shoes and surfaces hosted by the University of Calgary, accompanied by a published book of presented papers. Ned Frederick published the book *Sports Shoes and Playing Surfaces – Biomechanical Aspects* in 1985, and Calgary hosted a further symposium in 1988, this time focused only on sports surfaces. Some years later in 2003 Calgary held the Third Symposium on Sports Surfaces, and in 2005 the network SportSURF (Sports Surfaces Forum) was founded. Scientific and engineering interest in sports surfaces has led to the development of organisations such as the International Association for Sports Surfaces (ISSS) and the Sports Turf Research Institute (STRI), and the publication of several research and review papers in the field. However, time has passed without the collection of scientific and engineering progress in the form of a book.

This current book aims to provide an up-to-date evaluation of current thinking, and practice to an extent, and includes aspects of surface types and technologies, standards and testing, player movement and safety, user performance, and future directions for the industry and research. As new information emerges and new research is performed, some of the facts and figures may become a little dated but the basic principles and underpinning science are expected to have currency for the next 30 years and beyond.

Sharon Dixon, Paul Fleming, Iain James and Matt Carré

# Acknowledgements

The authors would like to acknowledge the contribution of Dr Steph Forrester (Senior Lecturer, Mechanical and Manufacturing Engineering, Loughborough University) in providing valuable feedback on Chapters 4 and 7 during the writing of this book.

The authors would also like to acknowledge the following for contributions made to the materials provided in the book: The Sports and Play Construction Association (SAPCA); Labosport (UK) Ltd; Sport England.

# Abbreviations

| | |
|---|---|
| AA | Artificial Athlete |
| AAA | Advanced Artificial Athlete |
| ACL | Anterior Cruciate Ligament |
| AFL | Australian Football League |
| AGP | Artificial Grass Soccer Pitch |
| ASTM | American Society for Testing and Materials |
| BS | British Standard |
| BW | Bodyweights |
| CE | European Conformity/European Community |
| ECB | England and Wales Cricket Board |
| EILLP | Exercise Induced Lower Leg Pain |
| EMG | Electromyography |
| EN | European Standard |
| EPDM | Ethylene Propylene Diene Monomer |
| EVA | Ethylene Vinyl Acetate |
| FIFA | Federation of International Football Associations |
| FIH | International Federation of Hockey (field hockey) |
| FPC | Factory Construction Control |
| FQC | Football Quality Concept |
| FR | Force Reduction (%), a measure of the relative shock-absorbency of a surface compared to concrete. A low FR = a harder surface, concrete = 0 per cent |
| GRF | Ground Reaction Force |
| IAAF | International Association of Athletics Federations |
| IGB | International Governing Body |
| ISO | International Organisation for Standardisation |
| ISSS | International Association of Sports Surface Sciences |
| ITF | International Tennis Federation |
| MTP | Metatarsal-Phalangeal |
| MUGA | Multi-Use Games Area |
| NGB | National Governing Body |

| | |
|---|---|
| QA | Quality Assurance (system to provide consistency in testing methods and construction processes) |
| QC | Quality Concept (a process of quality assuring a product and installation) |
| QC | Quality Control (usually factory control of manufacture) |
| Ra | Measure of surface roughness |
| RAPRA | The Rubber and Plastics Research Association Technology Ltd. |
| RFL | Rugby Football League |
| SBR | Styrene-Butadiene Rubber |
| STRI | Sports Turf Research Institute |
| TPE | Thermoplastic Elastomere |
| UEFA | Union of European Football Associations |
| USGA | United States Golf Association |
| WR | World Rugby |

Chapter 1

# Introduction

## History and development of sports surfaces

*Sharon Dixon, Paul Fleming, Iain James and Matt Carré*

### Introduction

This chapter introduces the subject of sports surfaces and outlines the themes introduced in the book. Examples are used to illustrate different types of sports surface, highlighting key historical developments. A need for standardisation and testing is stressed, including the incorporation of tests with players. The importance of research is highlighted, and the role of natural turf surfaces is outlined.

### What is a sports surface?

The answer to this question can be quite different depending on whether you are a participant, maintenance provider (grounds manager, greenkeeper), manufacturer, installer, spectator or researcher. Many sports that are still extremely popular today have origins that date back many years, when surfaces would typically have been local fields and common open spaces. More modern forms of these sports are played on specially prepared surfaces, specifically designed for the game requirements, but still have a long history; international cricket test matches began in 1844, international Davis Cup matches for tennis have been held since 1900, field hockey has been included as a modern Olympic event since 1908 and the dimensions of an association football rules pitch were laid out in 1863.

The range of surfaces used for sports participation today appears unlimited. Surfaces include grass, wood, concrete, acrylic, rubber, carpet, clay, cinder, soil, foam, asphalt and sand (often in combination with each other). Since the original development of sports, there have been huge advances in natural surface preparation (e.g. drainage systems, soil composition, grass cultivation, cutting and rolling technology), and more recently technological leaps forward in the development of artificial surfaces and hybrid systems (polymer fibre carpets, sand-based and rubber-based systems, grass fibre reinforcement).

Chapter 2 describes in detail these advances in surface technology and construction. These changes have made huge differences to the access to, enjoyment of and even style of play, perhaps most noticeably in field hockey.

## The rise of artificial surfaces

A desire to provide consistent surfaces to improve elite sports performance, together with the development of strategies to increase sports participation, has led to the development and increased usage of artificial sports surfaces, outlined in Chapter 2. Synthetic running tracks and artificial turf provide two examples. Running tracks have been developed to allow optimal performance by minimising the influence of weather conditions on the interaction with the surface – hence the term 'all-weather' track. Early tracks were cinder, clay or grass, meaning that weather had a significant influence on their performance. The first artificial running surface is thought to have been a warm-up track constructed for the 1956 Summer Olympics in Melbourne, Australia, made from a mix of asphalt and rubber. Polyurethane 'Tartan' track surfaces were developed in the 1960s by the company 3M. The 1968 Summer Olympics in Mexico saw the first synthetic track being used for an Olympics. In contrast to this focus on elite sports performance, in the mid-1960s the Ford Foundation (www.fordfoundation.org), in an effort to improve the fitness of young people, challenged Monsanto Industries to develop an urban sports surface suitable for use in schools. This led to the development of the first artificial turf surface for sports, first installed at a school in Rhode Island in 1964. The same surface was subsequently installed at the Houston Astrodome in 1966, home of the Houston Astros baseball and American football teams. This led to the name 'astroturf', still commonly used as a generic term for synthetic turf today. Synthetic turf surfaces have been adopted widely, with the main motivation being to provide a surface that allows repeated use in all weathers with limited maintenance, thus improving the availability of the playing surface to a greater and wider population.

A common focus when applying synthetic materials to the development of sports surfaces has been on providing suitable surfaces for safe performance at an optimal level. History demonstrates that the initial applications of synthetic materials in sports surface development were not always successful in achieving these aims. For example, the early use of artificial pitches in American football was associated with injuries such as abrasions and 'turf toe', while the initial use of these surfaces in soccer was also associated with marked changes in performance requirements as a result of both shoe–surface and ball–surface interactions (Dixon, Batt and Collop, 1999).

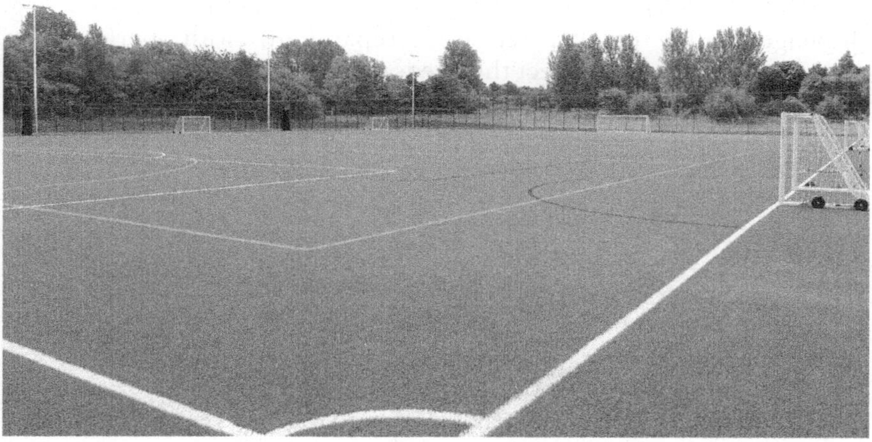

*Figure 1.1* An example of a community 3G synthetic turf surface © Iain James, 2014.

More recently, sports surface research and technological advances have led to the development of artificial surfaces that are more acceptable to sports participants, either because they are considered to adequately reproduce the playing conditions of natural turf (e.g. soccer), or the changes as a result of using the surface are considered to enhance the sport (e.g. track and field athletics, field hockey). This acceptance has also led to a large increase in availability of artificial surfaces for recreational sports participation (Figure 1.1). The commitment to increased use of these surfaces is demonstrated by the English Football Foundation investment of £31 million, funded by the English Football Association (FA), the English Football Premier League and the UK Government, in the development of facilities for recreational football, primarily focused on the installation of third-generation football turf pitches (Football Association, 2014). At the elite level, artificial surfaces are becoming increasingly accepted by sports governing bodies, as demonstrated by: the English FA approving their use for any FA Cup matches from 2014–2015; most venues for the FIFA Women's Soccer World Cup 2015 being artificial turf; and recently their introduction to premiership rugby union in the UK at Saracens and Newcastle Falcons.

## Standards and control for playing performance

An increase in the use of artificial systems has also contributed to a rise in the standardisation and testing of surfaces. Chapter 3 provides detail on the functional and performance-related requirements of quality assurance for sports surface systems, common test procedures and apparatus. The testing of surfaces has combined the types of standard protocols that have stemmed from the civil engineering industry (e.g. drainage, build quality, surface preparation) with performance measures, developed to meet the needs of customers, players and sports governing bodies (e.g. ball roll, ball bounce and surface comfort and grip). Standards are updated as new knowledge emerges, particularly related to safety and durability.

## Player interaction with surfaces

Casual participation sports can take place on almost any available surface – for example football (soccer) can be seen being played on various surfaces around the world including roads (asphalt), sand, grass, soil, cinder and synthetic grass.

Individuals are able to adapt their play to the different surfaces, both in terms of the player–surface interaction and the movement of the ball on the surface. While this requirement for adaptation does influence the game, this level of freedom can add to the variety and enjoyment. However, it is acknowledged that there are both injury and performance implications when selecting a surface for a particular sport. Chapters 4 and 5, respectively, discuss the role of sports surfaces in influencing injury risk and performance.

Sports surfaces have changed phenomenally since the early days of competitive sport. For outdoor sports, the properties of these surfaces would have been determined primarily by the weather conditions, with harder natural surfaces in dry, warm climates and soft, often muddy surfaces in wetter locations. Participants would have adapted to the conditions, typically using their past experience of the conditions to adjust their movement patterns to allow optimal performance regardless of the surface conditions – this would have been an accepted part of the sport. Tennis is a modern example of the need for player adaptation, with high-profile international tournaments being played on three very different surfaces: 'hardcourts' (a relatively stiff surface utilising a top surface of acrylic paint mixed with silica particles) used at the Australian and US Open; 'clay' (an unbound surface with a top layer of particles free to move, that requires sweeping and watering for preparation) used at the French Open; and 'grass' (a natural surface that requires professional preparation and can be affected by the elements, as well as being worn over the duration of a tournament) used at Wimbledon. In recent years there have also been trends for elite tennis players to change their style of movement, for instance an increasing tendency to slide on hardcourts, in a similar style to that typical on clay. An improved understanding of player response to different surfaces and the factors that govern this response can be used to inform the development of safe surfaces for optimal performance.

## Research

A need to understand the role of different parameters and components (e.g. for long pile soccer and rugby 3G systems, the carpet, in-fill, and shockpad) in achieving high quality safe surfaces has stimulated much research, aiming to better understand the complex player and equipment interactions that occur. Chapters 6 and 7, respectively, discuss the mechanical and biomechanical considerations required to improve understanding of the interaction between the player and the surface.

Research into sports surfaces has focused on both performance and injury risk requirements. The development of a scientific interest in sports surfaces during the 1980s led to an International Symposium on Biomechanical Aspects of Sports Shoes and Playing Surfaces hosted by the University of Calgary in 1983. Here 37 researchers contributed to 21 papers presented on sports footwear and playing surfaces (Nigg and Kerr, 1983). In one of these papers, Benno Nigg highlighted that prior to 1970 there were just eight research publications on sports footwear and playing surfaces, with this increasing to 35 publications in this field during the 1970s. A Medline search performed in April 2014 considering papers published between 2004 and 2014, using ['sports and shoes' or 'playing surfaces'] returned 359 hits. The first symposium on sports shoes and playing surfaces was followed by a second focused solely on sports surfaces in 1988. Around the same time as the first symposium, the book *Sport Shoes and Playing Surfaces – Biomechanical Properties*, edited by Ned Frederick (1984), was published. In the preface, the timeliness of the book is highlighted, with reference to the 'discovery' at this time that shoes and surfaces can make a difference to the biomechanics of the performer. The book describes a series of articles on subjects including friction characteristics of playing surfaces, functional standards for playing surfaces, and the influence of track compliance on running. In 2003, the Third Symposium on Sports Surfaces took place in Calgary, attended by a wide audience of sports scientists, engineers and practitioners. Formed in 2005, the network SportSURF has provided a forum for sports surface research, with more than 300 members across academia and industry. This organisation has hosted several technical seminars and two international conferences (http://sportsurf.lboro.ac.uk). Scientific and engineering interest has also led to the development of organisations such as the International Association for Sport Surface Sciences (ISSS).

## Natural turf

Despite the described rise in use of artificial sports surfaces, natural turf surfaces remain an important feature of many sports, both at the elite level (Figure 1.2) and in recreational community sport (Figure 1.3). Huge advances have been made in recent times in the provision of high-quality natural surfaces, which will remain the elite standard for many sports, and will always have a role in sports, particularly those that utilise large playing areas. Chapter 8 includes detail on developments in natural turf provision aimed at facilitating the quality and reliability of the surface, particularly in wet conditions.

Natural turf surfaces are more widely available. In 2012, Sport England's database of community sports facilities in England included just under 2,000 synthetic turf pitches for football and field hockey in England, primarily in urban locations. The same database catalogues 12,300 full-sized (and 8,000 junior) natural turf football pitches, with a much wider geographical spread into smaller-sized communities. Often sports participation relies on natural turf facilities that require investment in drainage and in routine maintenance to allow year-round usage, particularly in wet weather. Facilities such as those in Figure 1.3 are

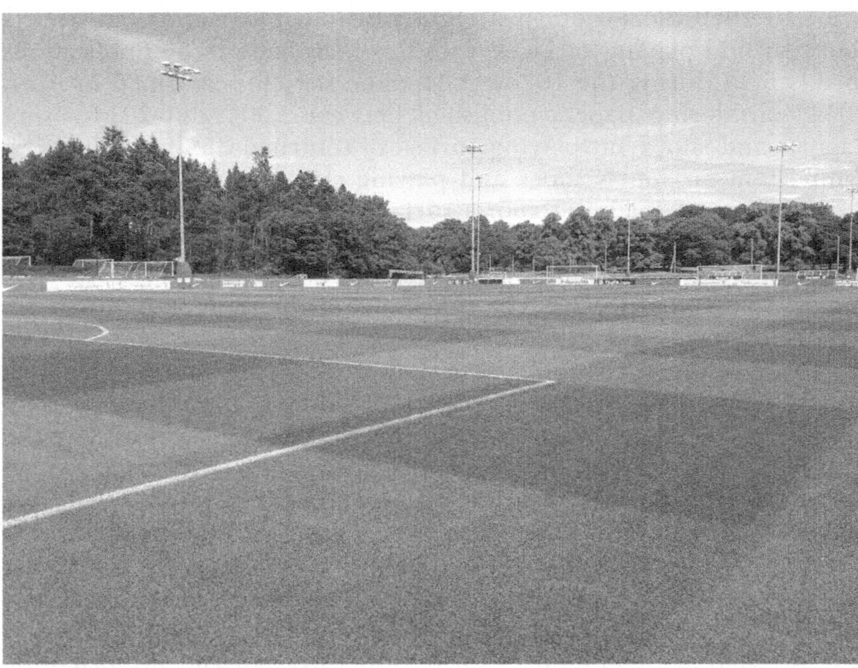

*Figure 1.2* The elite-level hybrid natural turf surface at the English FA's National Football Centre, St George's Park © Iain James, 2014.

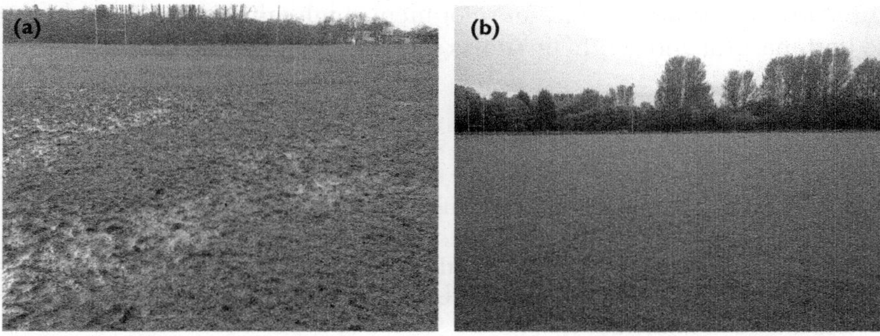


*Figure 1.3* Example of an improved natural turf surface: (a) before drainage; (b) immediately following drainage and improvement © TGMS Ltd, 2014.

critical for community participation, but are unplayable in prolonged wet conditions unless they are drained and well-maintained. Chapter 8 considers developments in natural turf and how these surfaces can be optimised for improved performance and for continued use in adverse weather conditions.

## A multidisciplinary subject

Research, development, design and control of sports surfaces are carried out by many disciplines and by professionals and experts from many different backgrounds. Consequently, the language used to describe certain aspects of interest can vary widely, across disciplines and around the world. We have provided a glossary which we hope will aid readers from different fields by defining terms such as 'ground reaction force', 'soil shear strength' and 'shoe–surface traction' and help to put them into their appropriate context.

## Conclusion

The following chapters set out to cover many of the issues raised in this chapter and have been written by researchers from different relevant fields, often in combination. The chapters can also be read in isolation, for readers who are interested in a specific aspect of sports surfaces. Chapters provide examples from different sports owing to the focus of different research areas and technological developments. Research and development continues to drive improvement of sports surfaces and, hopefully, can allow increased, safe, enjoyable and competitive participation in sport for the improved health and wellbeing of society in the future. The final chapter of this book (Chapter 9) considers future directions for sports surface development, highlighting aspects relevant to both natural and synthetic sports surfaces.

## References

Dixon, S. J., Batt, M. E. and Collop, A. C. (1999) 'Artificial playing surfaces research: A review of medical, engineering and biomechanical aspects', *International Journal of Sports Medicine*, 20: 209–218.

Football Association (2014) www.thefa.com/news/thefa/2014/oct/grassroots-projects-get-7m-from-the--premier-league-and-the-fa-facilities-fund--071014. Retrieved 9 October 2014.

Frederick, E. C. (ed.) (1984) *Sports Shoes and Playing Surfaces*. Champaign, IL: Human Kinetics.

Nigg, B. M. and Kerr, B. A. (eds) (1983) *Biomechanical Aspects of Sport Shoes and Playing Surfaces*. Calgary: University Printing.

Chapter 2

# Surface classification, function, construction and maintenance

*Iain James*

## Introduction

Sports surfaces vary between sports and within sports, reflecting the performance requirements of the surface and the properties of the different materials and combinations of materials that are used to construct the surface. Classifying sports surfaces allows an understanding to be formed of how a particular sports surface is likely to behave, how it will wear and how it needs to be maintained to ensure that it meets the required performance specification for the particular sport being played. The most obvious approach to classifying sports surfaces is by the sport being played, e.g. a 'football pitch', a 'tennis court', a 'golf course' or an 'athletics track'. This makes sense because it is often the sport that defines the performance requirements such as smooth ball roll and good grip (traction) for a football pitch, but good ball bounce and pace for a tennis court. However there can be significant variation within a sport. Consider the range of court surfaces used in tennis. As highlighted in Chapter 1, the four 'major' championships include two types of hard court (Australian Open and US Open), clay (French Open) and natural turf (Wimbledon). The challenge for classifying surfaces by sport comes when a surface is to be used for a number of different sports, whether it is in an elite sports stadium or a recreational playing field. Examples of this include synthetic turf surfaces used for both hockey and football, football stadia used to play rugby union, and use of cricket grounds in Australia for Australian football. It is therefore necessary to classify surfaces by both sport and construction type.

It is often difficult to determine the factors responsible for a particular sports surface design. Sports surface design is a combination of a number of factors including:

- **Playing rules and regulations.** Playing rules and regulations affect both the design and maintenance of a sports surface in terms of both the performance and risk of injury for a surface. Note that playing rules and regulations can also be defined by the surface design.

- **Innovations in style or technique of play.** An example would be the introduction of over-arm bowling into cricket, which then meant that ball bounce characteristics became more critical and made greater demands on the ball bounce performance of the surface leading ultimately to the use of imported clay soils.
- **Availability of resources.** Where space, materials, finances or maintenance inputs are limited this has fostered the development of surfaces that are more resistant to wear and require less materials for maintenance. An example would be the development of polymeric running tracks or the use of synthetic turf in inner cities.
- **Product innovation.** There is constant innovation in materials, construction systems and maintenance equipment to improve the performance and safety of sports surfaces. An example would be the Desso Grassmaster system which uses synthetic turf fibres to improve the resilience of natural turf football and rugby pitches.
- **Injury reduction.** Some innovation in sports surface design is driven by injury reduction, commonly the reduction of stiffness or hardness and either the increase or reduction of grip (traction) to limits set as 'safe' levels for players.
- **Governing body sports surface performance requirements/ standards.** It is increasingly common for both international and national sports governing bodies to specify laboratory and in-field test methods and accreditation criteria/benchmarks. An example would be the FIFA Quality Concept for synthetic turf surfaces used in football (soccer), which benchmarked high-quality natural turf and set upper and lower limits for a range of test parameters which must be met for a particular pitch to be designated as meeting either a one-star or two-star standard. Pitches achieving the two-star standard can be used in the qualification rounds of the FIFA World Cup.
- **Environmental adaptations and requirements.** Environmental conditions such as climate can drive the design and selection of sports surface. For example the use of synthetic turf surfaces for football is common in northern European countries where significant snowfall and permafrost can limit the use of natural turf. Design adaptation can also occur due to concerns over environmental impact. There is an identified need to increase the recycling of synthetic turf systems at end of life and this is driving modern synthetic turf system design.
- **Participation and income generation.** Access to safe, sustainable and performance sports surfaces helps to encourage and sustain participation in sport, and to provide essential income generation to support the development of the sports facility and club. Where fixtures and events are routinely cancelled due to poor weather or damage from excessive use, participation and financial sustainability will be limited.

- **Spectator and viewer requirements.** This is an increasingly common driver for development in elite sport whereby fixture cancellation or visually poor surfaces can adversely affect spectator and viewer experience and lead to disgruntled broadcasters and reduced television and radio income.

Modern sports surface development is driven by these factors. It is important to recognise that sports surfaces wear and degrade with use and environmental exposure. The rate of wear and degradation depends on the intensity of use, the resistance of materials to wear and the severity of the environment. This in turn affects the quantity and frequency of maintenance required to provide a sustainable and safe provision of sport use at the required level of performance. Routine, effective maintenance is an essential requirement for all sports surfaces but is particularly significant in natural turf systems. Without maintenance, high-performing facilities can rapidly become irreversibly unusable; ultimately this will require costly replacement to avoid the loss of an asset.

It is evident that there are many design and operational factors that are critical for sports surface performance and safety. These factors will be considered in detail for a range of surface systems throughout this chapter as sports surfaces are characterised by both sport and construction type.

## Surfaces for different types of football

In this section surfaces for a range of football codes are considered including association football (soccer), rugby football (Union and League), Australian football, Gaelic football and American football.

### *Natural turf*

Natural turf 'fields' were the original surface for many sports and in particular for football. The modern natural turf football pitch is very different from traditional surfaces which were animal pastures and other grassed areas, mown to produce playing fields for sport.

Natural turf surfaces can provide excellent playing characteristics for football offering a balance between ball–surface and player–surface interactions due to the effect of the grass plant and the underlying soil (Figure 2.1). The role of the grass plant is to reinforce the soil which would otherwise be damaged more easily. The grass also affects player underfoot grip (termed 'traction'), the hardness of a surface and reduces player–surface and ball–surface friction. However the grass plant is organic, it must receive sufficient water, air, light and nutrients to sustain growth and recover from wear. Soil–plant–environment interactions

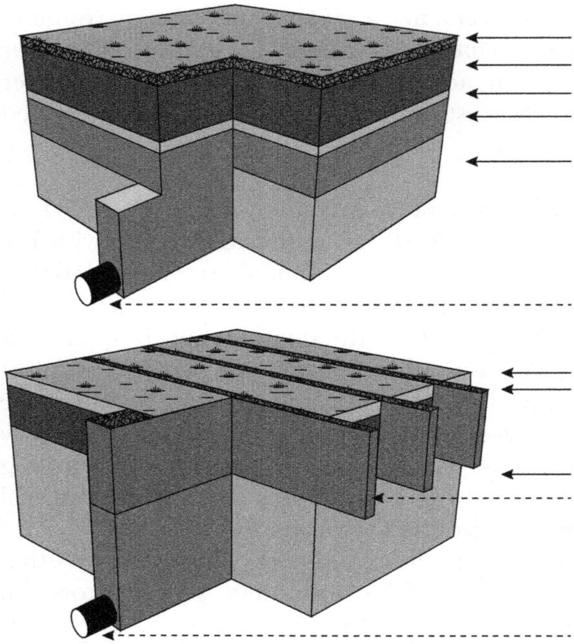


*Figure 2.1* Cross-sections of two types of natural turf construction. Top: a 'sand rootzone carpet' commonly used in football stadia. Bottom: a 'sand bypass' drainage system of more closely spaced lateral drains intersected with sand grooves or slits that connect directly to the surface to allow water to reach the subsurface drainage rapidly.

are essential in determining the performance and durability of natural turf surfaces. These interactions are discussed in more detail in Chapter 8 but the key requirement for natural turf at recreational and elite level is for effective drainage. This is because the shear strength of soils and the strength of the grass plant decreases as the soil becomes very wet, and a wet surface is easily damaged. Modern elite natural turf football surfaces are built using high sand content soils that drain easily into closely spaced sub-surface drains. In fact they are so free-draining they commonly have to be irrigated to provide enough water for the plant to survive. However they have much greater wear resistances than traditional natural turf surfaces constructed from natural soils, which are commonly poorly draining.

An advantage of natural turf is that given sufficient light, water and nutrients the plant will regenerate following stress and wear. The cut height of the grass is traditionally varied in sport, being lower for association football (20–25 mm) to reduce drag on the ball and longer in sports such as rugby football (35–50 mm) to increase wear resistance and reduce the impact on players. The frequency of cutting will depend on how quickly the grass is growing (greatest during late spring and early autumn at temperate latitudes). High-performance natural turf surfaces are high maintenance, requiring irrigation, fertiliser, pesticides and even supplementary growth lighting in some stadia. Natural turf surfaces are commonly spatially and temporally variable (see Chapter 8). In the elite stadium environment sources of variation are caused by differential shading from stands and variations in wear patterns from different sports. In the recreational environment, spatial variation can also be caused by variation in soil type, drainage, surface levels and lack of maintenance. All natural turf surfaces are subject to temporal variation due to environmental factors and in particular precipitation and temperature. This has been overcome in a few stadia worldwide that use a range of technologies to cover the stadium roof during play – these include whole pitches that can move in and out of stadia, stadia with retractable roofs and even a stadium with a fixed transparent roof (Dunedin, New Zealand).

Such extraordinary environmental engineering occurs because natural turf remains the preferred surface for all football codes, save perhaps for American football. With limited mowing a natural turf sports surface can provide a relatively low-cost facility for limited frequency of use at the recreational level and with significant inputs of time, money and natural resources it can provide the ultimate elite surface for football of all types. The limitations of natural turf (low wear resistance/carrying capacity, and high maintenance costs) have however led to the development of synthetic alternatives.

### *Synthetic turf*

Synthetic turf surfaces were originally developed in the 1960s with the first-generation, short-pile nylon surfaces providing greater wear resistance but reduced performance and higher player injury incidence than natural turf. Nylon surfaces were high friction and caused abrasions as well as a range of injuries related to surface hardness. A second generation of synthetic surfaces was developed in the 1970s and 1980s (Figure 2.2). These comprised a longer pile of 20–25 mm of polypropylene fibres tufted or woven into a backing material and then filled with rounded sand to keep the fibres vertical. This carpet was laid over a rubber shockpad, overlying a tarmacadam and angular stone base. These surfaces became extremely popular for both recreational use and elite-stadium use. They were widely used in American football where players are protected from abrasion by their clothing and the ball is predominantly carried or thrown, with little interaction with the surface. They were also used in elite soccer in England at clubs such as Oldham Athletic and

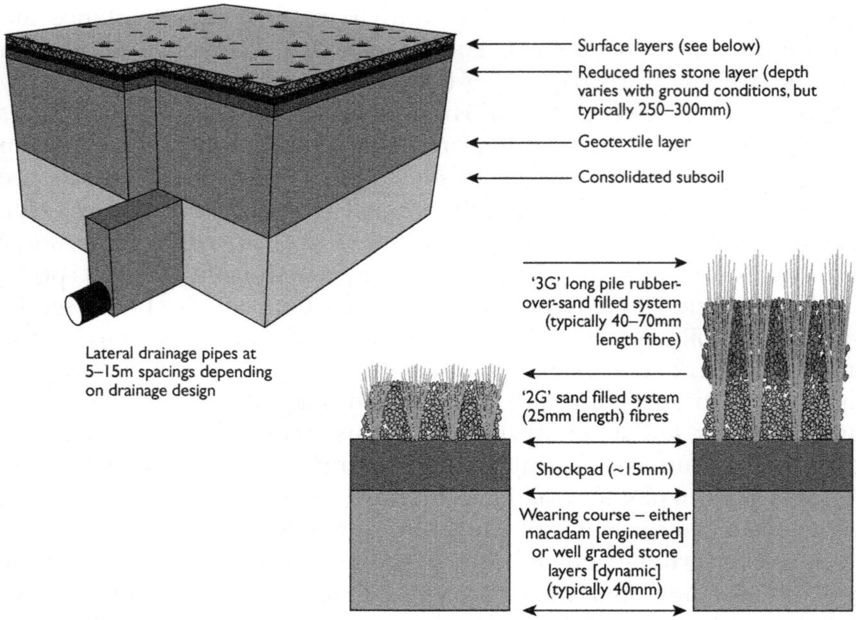


*Figure 2.2* Typical construction profiles for synthetic turf surfaces. The detail shows how the surface layers differ with longer pile and rubber infill found in modern third-generation (3G) surfaces used in football, when compared with older second-generation (2G) surfaces.

Luton Town but were eventually banned in the 1980s due to poor playability – in particular high ball bounce, high abrasion risk and concerns over unfair home advantage.

The 1990s saw the development of a third generation of synthetic turf surface with longer pile length (typically 40–90 mm) and a combination of sand and rubber granules used as infill (Figure 2.2). Third-generation synthetic turf has been widely accepted as a more suitable surface for not only association football but also rugby football and American and Australian football, with surfaces used around the world for national and international competitions. UEFA and then FIFA have led the way in developing playing performance and safety standards for third-generation turf surfaces, with FIFA sanctioning their use in World Cup qualifying tournaments and the Women's World Cup Finals, and their use in national leagues across Europe. There is still resistance to their use in the English Men's Premier League (Tier 1), primarily due to historical objections to the use of second-generation turf and a concern over injury risk, but the use of third-generation synthetic turf is being considered for lower leagues (Tiers 2–4), and it is already in competition use below this level.

Synthetic turf has a number of key advantages over natural turf. It is more resistant to wear and has a greater carrying capacity, making it ideal for intensive community sport. Synthetic turf is inorganic and does not require light or irrigation and is freely draining – it can therefore be used in shaded stadia and indoors. While its maintenance requirement is lower than high-specification natural turf, synthetic turf systems are not maintenance free and require routine brushing and cleaning to maintain performance levels and keep drainage rates high (James and McLeod, 2010; Fleming, 2011). Maintenance costs per hour of use are significantly lower than for natural turf, which makes them attractive for income generation.

Third-generation synthetic turf describes a range of systems with varying pile lengths, pile materials, production methods, infill materials and construction profiles. Shorter pile lengths of 40 mm are suitable for football and lower-level field hockey. Longer pile lengths are used for football (ca 60 mm) and even longer for rugby (90 mm) – this allows for more infill and greater shock absorbency, critical for reducing the risk of injury in contact sports such as rugby, American and Australian football. World Rugby has a performance quality standard similar to that of FIFA but with a greater shock absorbency and a separate head impact criterion that must be met for a surface to be approved for play in rugby union. In the 2012 Rugby League 'Super League' Widnes Vikings were the first UK Tier 1 rugby side to use a 60 mm pile, sand-rubber infill surface in their stadium. This was followed in 2013 by the English Premiership Rugby Union side Saracens.

Construction profiles are typically an engineered system comprising a drainage system for surface water, angular stone sub-base and tarmacadam wearing courses, with a shock pad beneath the carpet which is then filled with sand and granulated rubber. In order to reduce construction costs the tarmacadam layer is not utilised in a 'dynamic base' system, but concerns have been raised about whether this approach reduces the lifespan of the surface. Synthetic turf surfaces do wear over time and have a typical replacement period of eight to ten years depending on maintenance and intensity of use – following this the 'carpet' is removed and replaced. It is difficult to recycle the removed carpet due to the combination of materials that are not easily separated – improved recycling of materials at end of life is a sustainability challenge for the industry to solve.

The performance of longer-pile third-generation synthetic turf systems is much improved and is closer to that of natural turf but product/system development is still required to manage the balance between player–surface and ball–surface interactions over a longer period of use (surfaces tend to become harder over time, resulting in greater ball bounce and reduced player comfort). With increasing use in lower-level competitions and the financial advantages of synthetic turf over natural turf, the synthetic turf surface is likely to become more common in football sports.

## Surfaces for tennis

Lawn tennis is played on a range of surface types which have different playing characteristics, which mean that players have to adapt their playing style and movement to adjust to different player grip (traction) and ball–surface interactions. Tennis courts are 23.78 m (78 ft) long and 10.97 m (36 ft) wide (including doubles tramlines). Different surfaces exist because of different climates, maintenance requirements and traditions. The following sections look at three principal types – the grass court, the clay court and the hard court.

### *Grass/artificial grass courts*

Grass is the original surface for lawn tennis (as suggested by the name) and is characterised by fast pace and low bounce. Grass tennis courts are constructed on heavily compacted clay loam soil over a firm sub-base of compacted soil or stone. Grass is seeded into the soil and maintained at a low cutting height to provide a hard, fast surface for ball rebound. Grass was used for both the Australian Open (until 1988) and the US Open (until 1975) but the only one of the four major tournaments to still use grass is the Wimbledon Championships in England. Even in England, only 7 per cent of tennis courts are grass courts and a number of these are at Wimbledon or at facilities hosting warm-up or qualifying tournaments for Wimbledon. The reason for reduced numbers of grass courts is because they are extremely sensitive to weather and cannot be played on when wet – this means that play has to be suspended and the court either covered or allowed to dry before it is used again, otherwise it will become damaged by players and players will slip during play. Grass courts are not suitable for winter use because the grass is dormant and will not recover from wear. Grass courts are relatively high maintenance compared to other surfaces because they need to be mown, rolled and irrigated frequently and can require significant applications of fertiliser and pesticide. Synthetic turf provides a lower-maintenance alternative compared to grass but with different player and ball–surface interactions; 17 per cent of English tennis courts are synthetic turf.

### *Clay/artificial clay courts*

Original clay tennis courts were made from clay soil/rock that was compacted to form a surface that was comfortable to play on and required less maintenance than a grass court but that could not be played on when wet or used for a number of days after rainfall due to poor drainage. This meant that original clay courts were more suited to warmer, drier climates. The majority of modern clay surfaces are not actually formed from clay materials but crushed harder materials such as clay brick or basalt (igneous rock) which provide better drainage. This leads to a wide array of clay court types, often referred to by their colour. The red clay courts used in the French Open are formed from crushed clay brick but a range of 'colours' or different materials are used in Tour events leading up to the French Open major championship. The US Open used green coloured crushed (basalt) clay with a sub-surface irrigation system between 1975 and 1977 before switching to a hard-court surface. Clay surfaces provide a higher, slower ball bounce that gives the player more time to play a return shot, making it harder to hit a winner and more likely that points are decided on player error. This results in longer rallies than on grass courts. Clay surfaces allow the player to slide more than on other surface types and consequently players need time to adapt to the surface. This issue is discussed further in Chapters 4 and 7.

Clay courts are constructed over a piped drainage system with a compacted stone base. The clay profile is built up above the stone base. Although clay courts do not require mowing and fertiliser they do require frequent rolling to maintain surface levels and irrigation to maintain cohesion of the surface to prevent cracking and break-up. Therefore clay tennis courts should not be considered as low maintenance and are not suitable where water availability is restricted. The moist surface does lead to staining of footwear and clothes. Clay surfaces are uncommon in England (3 per cent) but very popular in France, Spain and warmer climates.

### *Hard courts (acrylic, asphalt)*

The term 'hard court' covers a range of surfaces such as acrylic, asphalt and concrete laid over an aggregate stone base to form a surface that is more rigid and does not deform as much as clay or grass surfaces. The majority of tennis courts are hard courts as they have much lower maintenance and much higher durability than grass or clay courts (for example, 71 per cent of English tennis courts are hard courts). They can also be used in wet conditions, provided that the player can maintain grip (traction). Two of the major tournaments are played on hard courts. The US Open is played on an acrylic resin surface that is painted onto a styrene-butadiene rubber (SBR) shock-absorbing layer overlying a stone base. The Australian Open uses a similar system over an ethylene propylene diene monomer (M-class) rubber (EPDM) layer. Both these surfaces have a shock-absorbing layer but acrylic surface finishes can be painted directly onto asphalt or concrete – but these surfaces will be harder providing lower shock-absorbency for the player. The majority of hard court tennis courts are of this type without a shock-absorbent layer. The pace and bounce of the court can be modified by the shock-absorbing layer and by the quantity, size and shape of the sand used in the paint. Ball rebound height is increased and pace reduced as ball–surface friction increases as the sand content or size is increased. Hard court pace is faster than clay but not as fast as grass. Hard court tennis surfaces are ideal for community/recreational sport due to their low maintenance requirement and suitability to a range of climates. Due to their low permeability they can result in greater rainfall runoff than the other court types and this should be considered in the management of surface water and flooding.

### *Performance specification*

While variation among surface types is expected, the International Tennis Federation provides a classification system for court pace (in terms of ball speed) for comparison of courts (ITF, 2012). This is described in more detail in Chapter 3.

## Athletics

### *Outdoor athletics surfaces*

Like tennis and so many other sports, the original surface for athletics running tracks was grass, which is still used at a recreational level. Grass surfaces were replaced by lower-maintenance unbound mineral surfaces such as the cinder (crushed volcanic rock) Iffley Road track in Oxford where Roger Bannister ran the first sub-four minute mile. These surfaces have almost universally been replaced by synthetic surfaces of different types to provide a low-maintenance, consistent, high-performance surface for athletics. It should be noted that although the modern athletics track and associated run-up and take-off areas are synthetic, the majority of the infield remains natural grass where javelins, shots, discuses and hammers land.

The International Association of Athletics Federations (IAAF) specify key performance characteristics for athletics tracks (IAAF, 2008). A grade of up to 1 per cent fall from the outside to the inside of the track is allowed to assist with shedding water but inclination should not exceed 0.1 per cent downwards in the direction of running to prevent athletes being given an unfair advantage from one track to the next when setting world records. The majority of high-performance outdoor tracks are 8–9 lane, 400 m tracks with a single radius of curvature (optimum of 36.50 m with straights of 84.39 m length). The dynamic mechanical properties of an athletics track need to balance the requirements of short-distance sprinters who desire a high-stiffness, low-deformation track that provides high-energy return, with middle- and long-distance runners who require a more compliant surface for comfort (see Chapters 4 and 5). Surface friction is also a key parameter to allow athletes to achieve sufficient but not excess grip (traction), with or without spiked footwear (see Chapters 5 and 6).

Synthetic athletics tracks are either permeable over an asphalt and stone base, or impermeable over an asphalt or concrete-over-stone base. The finished surfaces are made from rubber or polyurethane or a mixture of the two. The surface used at all the Olympics from Barcelona (1992) to London (2012) was a prefabricated textured rubber surface. However, the majority of surfaces are actually mixed and cast on site using either polyurethane with a rubber crumb (granules) surface or resin-bound rubber crumb. Prefabricated tracks have the advantage of greater quality control as they are less dependent upon weather conditions during construction but they must be accurately assembled and bonded to the sub-base structure very carefully using specialist adhesives. The resin-bound rubber crumb surfaces have the advantage that they are porous and allow water to drain through the surface. Standing water on poorly constructed, ageing or poorly maintained surfaces can be a significant problem, particularly in high-wear areas such as high jump take-off areas and javelin runways. Synthetic tracks need regular maintenance to ensure that the running surface is even and that algae and other infestations are prevented from forming, particularly in wet areas.

### *Indoor athletics surfaces*

Indoor athletics tracks are 200 m with bends banked between 10 and 15 degrees, and an infield 60 m sprint straight. The construction method for the track depends on whether the track is a permanent installation in a dedicated facility. Design and construction of permanent installations are similar to outdoor tracks but dedicated facilities are rare because they are of single use. This inflexibility of use can be overcome by installing a hydraulic system to raise and lower the banking on the bends, allowing the facility to be used as a flat surface when not used for athletics. Alternatively, temporary or portable track systems can be used which are formed from plywood over a timber structure, which is then surfaced with a suitable synthetic surface. The design of portable surfaces must ensure uniform resilience throughout the track by spacing the framework carefully beneath the plywood surface. Framework spacing was the method used by McMahon and Greene to optimise the stiffness of the track at Harvard University in their seminal study of running in which an optimised track stiffness was associated with improved athlete performance (McMahon and Greene, 1979).

## Golf

Golf courses are almost universally natural turf but there are a range of different surface types within the golf course. Each of the 18 holes in a typical course starts at a 'tee' and ends on a 'green'. On Par 3 holes the ball is driven directly to the green. On Par 4 and 5 holes fairways provide a staged landing area for hitting the ball towards the green. On every hole the tee and the green are visited by every golfer and as a consequence are high-traffic areas demanding freely draining soils to limit the wear of the grass. This has led to the development of the sand construction golf green and tee which pioneered the use of high sand-content soils over gravels and piped drainage systems to increase hydraulic conductivity of water from the surface to drainage outfall while maintaining a smooth putting surface on the golf green or a firm tee for the initial drive. The USGA (United States Golf Association) specification for golf green construction closely specifies the particle sizes used for both the sand rootzone and the gravel drainage layer so that the surface is free draining but a water table is suspended above the gravel by capillary forces to help with plant growth. This specification is used worldwide but does require frequent irrigation and the use of large quantities of fertiliser. To achieve fast ball roll on golf greens the grass will be cut to below 5 mm in length, which places significant stress on the grass plant, increasing susceptibility to disease and an associated increase in pesticide use.

Fairways are much larger in area than greens and tees and are too expensive to construct and maintain using the same approach. Therefore they tend to be formed from native soils. Larger golf courses and golf courses in drier climates will irrigate fairways to maintain turf quality and consequently water use by golf courses can be significant. Ball–surface interaction on fairways is different from greens with the focus on ball bounce as well as roll. The hardness of fairways determines how quickly a ball will stop on impact. Harder fairways provide more of a challenge to the golfer because it is difficult to control ball landing but can provide extra length on a drive. The fairways and greens are surrounded by rough grasses which are maintained at a longer length to act as hazards to the golfer as they are more difficult to play a controlled shot from. Other hazards include sand bunkers and water courses which can double as irrigation storage.

The majority of innovation in surface design, grass breeding and agronomic practice in golf has been due to the high maintenance intensity and the economic return that results. Golf courses have an aesthetic appeal that is perhaps best characterised by the Augusta National course in Georgia, USA but also in the coastal links courses of Scotland, such as St Andrews. Around the highly manicured turf, golf courses can provide important environmental habitats and have a significant role in wildlife ecology. This has to be balanced against the intensive use of fertilisers, pesticides and water that is associated with high presentational and performance quality.

## Cricket

Like golf, cricket is predominantly played on natural turf. In cricket the focus is on the ball bounce between bowler and batter. A similar approach to grass-court tennis is used with heavily compacted clay loam and clay soils used to produce a compact surface with closely mown grass to ensure maximum pace and bounce from the impact of a hard leather ball being bowled at high speed. The heavily compacted clay area is limited to a central array of pitches known as a square. Surrounding the square, the outfield can be an additional hectare of natural turf which is formed from indigenous soil or in the case of some elite venues from sand over an intensive drainage scheme, analogous to a large golf green. On the square the emphasis is on the ball–surface interaction and players wear narrow metal spikes to penetrate the heavily compacted clay surface and achieve appropriate grip (traction). The surface is hard and the load on the legs of the bowler is high. In the outfield the emphasis is on ball roll, where a hard surface for fast ball roll can be detrimental to players diving to field the ball. The amount of clay in the pitch increases in drier climates where the soil will dry more quickly when wetted – this creates variation in pitch performance around the world. Cricket pitches are expected to vary from ground to ground and over time in a sport where a game can last from a few hours to five days. Cricket grounds were used in the development of Australian football which is played on the large oval outfield. To help reduce the risk of injury and to reduce the wear of pitches, the central square can be removed pitch by pitch and replaced with sand soil in some grounds in Australia and New Zealand. This is discussed further in Chapter 8.

## Field hockey

Field hockey is a sport that has embraced the adoption of synthetic surfaces to the extent that the majority of hockey is played on synthetic turf and only very occasionally on grass. The transition to synthetic turf in the 1970s meant that the game became faster as rolling resistance for the ball decreased. On grass the ball was lifted or hit into the air more because rolling resistance for the relatively small ball was high. Bounce was unpredictable and led players to play with an upright stick to counter any variation in bounce. On synthetic surfaces the ball can be passed over longer distances along the ground and the ball can be transferred from end to end more quickly. This made the game more dynamic and both player- and spectator-friendly. Both playing techniques and equipment have adapted to this more dynamic version of the sport.

Recreational/community-level hockey is played on second generation sand filled (20–25 mm pile, filled to surface with sand) or sand dressed (15–20 mm denser pile, filled 50–80 per cent with sand) synthetic turf. Elite-level hockey is played on 'water-based' synthetic surfaces, which are short pile with no infill but are irrigated to maintain a fast, low-bounce wet surface that is considered ideal for hockey. The water also helps to reduce the ball–fibre friction. Water consumption is significant however as the pitches are irrigated before the game and at half time to keep them wet. This has prompted the International Hockey Federation (FIH) to work with the synthetic turf industry since 2006 to develop a 'dry' or low-water equivalent surface for use in elite-level competition to reduce the environmental impact of hockey and to allow hockey to be played in environments where water is scarce. Hockey also faces another challenge as second-generation synthetic turf surfaces are replaced with longer-pile third-generation surfaces used for football. While a 40 mm pile can be used as an introduction to hockey it is not suitable for competitive play because the stick can get further under the ball causing it to lift more dangerously and the longer pile length slows ball roll – effectively reversing the development of hockey back towards the original game on grass.

## Multi-use sports halls

The surface system of indoor sports halls needs to provide the same key parameters of force reduction, deformation and friction for player safety and performance. There are additional factors that must be considered including surface colour (to help players spot balls, shuttlecocks etc.), surface reflectance (to limit glare from overhead lighting), suitable line markings, surfaces that are easy to clean and maintain, and have good resistance to wear. These requirements vary from sport to sport. Dedicated specialist venues can optimise these parameters for a particular sport, for example dedicated coil-sprung gymnastics floors, lower-friction badminton floors and the high level of force reduction with minimum deformation required for basketball. To achieve maximum usage and therefore maximum revenue generation and participation, most sports halls are multi-sport and in schools and universities are likely to serve further functions such as events, exams and assemblies. Multi-use sports halls need to reach a compromise that puts multi-sport performance first but offers flexibility and wear resistance.

Key design variables include the surface construction (defining the dynamic properties) and the surface finish (determining the friction and optical characteristics). The European Standard EN 14904:2006 describes four categories of flooring system:

1 Point elastic – deformation is restricted to the actual point where load is applied, for example rubber shock-absorbing layers over concrete with acrylic/polyeurathane paint finishes. Such surfaces have high vertical deformation and appear soft under foot.
2 Mixed elastic – thicker foam-backed surfaces that spread some of the deformation over a greater area than point elastic surfaces.
3 Area elastic – deformation is spread over a greater area, providing force reduction with reduced vertical deformation, which helps to protect players from fatigue and provides a more stable footing. Area elastic surfaces tend to be timber boarding over a framework of lateral wooden beams or elastomer-sprung wooden beams.
4 Combined elastic – these surfaces combine an area sprung timber subbase with a thin point elastic rubber/foam surface coating/finish to provide a compromise surface which is commonly used for multi-use sports floors.

Area elastic and combined elastic surfaces are the most common in multi-use sports halls as they provide a balance between dynamic properties, wear resistance, flexibility of use and ease of maintenance.

## Summary

It is evident that there is a wide range of both outdoor and indoor sports surfaces, a range that reflects the varied requirements for player–surface and ball–surface interactions in different sports. The majority of outdoor sports originally used natural turf surfaces but have adapted to include synthetic alternatives that reduce the maintenance requirement and increase the usage compared to natural turf equivalents. Natural turf remains a preferred surface in many outdoor sports due to playing characteristics in football or the economics of area in sports such as cricket and golf. In sports such as field hockey and athletics there has been an almost complete move towards synthetic surfaces and in tennis a wide range of surfaces provide a global variety to the sport reflected in its major championships. In indoor sports halls the requirements of different sports are concentrated into a small area that must provide a compromise which allows different sports to share a common facility that performs for their sport in comfort and safety.

The majority of sport surface systems can be characterised by a load bearing sub-base, a shock-absorbing or force-reducing mid-layer and a performance-surface layer. As population increases, and urbanisation and development increase the pressure on the availability of sports surfaces, intensification of greater use on a smaller area is driving the demand for more weather- and wear-resistant surfaces. A key theme for outdoor surfaces is that the impact of water on performance and drainage is critical. In engineered synthetic systems drainage is relatively straightforward to design; in natural turf/soil systems this is a greater challenge and is discussed further in Chapter 8. Increasing the drainage and permeability of surfaces can require additional attenuation to limit flood risk downstream. While most sports have sport-specific performance requirements for surfaces there is an increasing trend towards multi-use facilities. Key design challenges for the future will be how to develop surfaces that achieve performance standards across a range of sports while carrying greater usage, without detriment to the environment in manufacturing, construction or use (in terms of pollution, flood risk, greenhouse gas emissions and waste) or to the diversity of sports within a community. It is essential that sports surfaces provide economic, social and environmental sustainability.

## Key summary points

- There are a wide range of both outdoor and indoor sports surfaces, a range that reflects the varied requirements for player–surface and ball–surface interactions in different sports.
- Natural turf remains the most common outdoor surface but there is an increasing move towards synthetic turf surfaces for durability, reduced operating costs and performance – although these requirements vary with the sport.
- The majority of sports surface systems can be characterised by a load-bearing sub-base, a shock-absorbing or force-reducing mid-layer and a performance-surface layer.
- A key challenge for sports surfaces engineering in the future will be to produce surfaces that can maintain high performance under ever-increasing intensity of participation and use, from an ever-decreasing area. This is driven by increasing population and urbanisation and will require more efficient use of scarce resources such as minerals, water and oil in their manufacture and maintenance.
- Production of high-performance, safe sports surfaces requires a detailed understanding of the mechanisms of player and equipment interactions with surfaces. These interactions, behaviours and systems are discussed in the following chapters of this book.

## References

Fleming, P. (2011) 'Maintenance best practice and recent research', *Proceedings of the Institution of Mechanical Engineers, Part P, Journal of Sports Engineering and Technology*, 225(3): 159–170.

IAAF (2008) *Track and Field Facilities Manual*, 2008 edition. Monaco: International Association of Athletics Federations. ISBN 2-911469-37-2. Available from: www.iaaf.org/about-iaaf/documents/technical

ITF (2012) *International Tennis Federation Court Pace Classification Programme: Guide to Applying for ITF Classification*. Available from: www.itftennis.com/technical/apply/court-classification/itf-court-pace-classification.aspx
James, I. T. and McLeod, A. J. (2010) 'The effect of maintenance on the performance of sand-filled synthetic turf surfaces', *Sports Technology*, 3(1): 43–51.
McMahon, T. A. and Greene, P. R. (1979) 'The influence of track compliance on running', *Journal of Biomechanics*, 12, 893–904.

Chapter 3

# Mechanical testing and characterisation of sports surfaces

*Paul Fleming, Colin Young and Matt Carré*

## Introduction

Testing of sports surfaces relates to user safety and product approval. Recent changes through European harmonisation of national standards has led to a complex array of standards relating to product approval (including individual elements and the 'as constructed' whole surface system) and in situ testing requirements.

Governing bodies (national and international, NGBs and IGBs) of sport have, over the past ten years in particular, developed their own frameworks for quality assurance (QA) of artificial turf and with regard to the intended competition level for the sport and more general community use. The approach they have taken is primarily to protect the way the game is played and to decrease safety risks to the users. NGB/IGBs have specific compliance requirements for approving facilities, and for regulating products sold into the market as 'fit for purpose'. While there is some commonality in test methods and equipment, subtle and significant differences exist, usually where the sport involves balls or is primarily played indoors as opposed to outdoors.

The scope of the testing methods covered here is related to the scope of surfaces set out in Chapter 2, wherein the types of surfaces used for sport, aspects of their design and construction, and aftercare were considered. However, this chapter does not explicitly cover all these sports as many of the testing requirements are somewhat generic, and the guidance can be categorised for surfaces used indoors or outdoors, for natural turf or artificial turf, or for other sport-specific types of synthetic surfaces.

The performance requirements set out in NGB/IGB guidance forms a primary set of constraints in the development of new surfaces by the industry. These standardised test methods also form the benchmark for classifying and ranking surfaces in the commercial domain, and for describing the properties of many of the surface systems reported in research literature relating to sports surfaces.

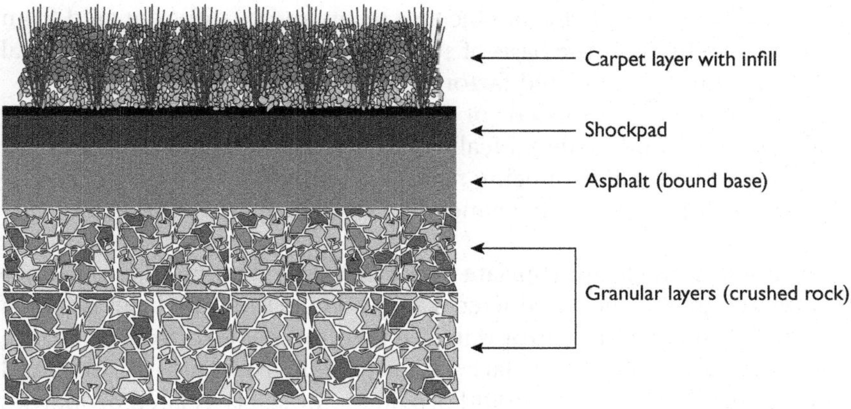


*Figure 3.1* Schematic of an artificial turf pitch system showing the layered structure. The carpet, infill and shockpad comprise the 'surface system', the layers beneath comprise the 'foundation' including the in situ soil (or fill) beneath the imported crushed rock.

This chapter provides a reference useful to many stakeholders with regard to the functional and performance-related requirements of quality assurance for sports surface systems, common test procedures and apparatus, and some current research thinking. The technical information and terminology are subsequently used in many of the later chapters, particularly Chapters 4, 5, 6, 7 and 9.

## General requirements of sports surfaces

A sports surface 'system' is usually composed of several components, and these are combined to provide the required functions and performance for the specific sport or a range of sports (multi-use). The advent of artificial surfaces has been observed to increase the range of systems and components on the market and in use, and generated a requirement to standardise both system performance requirements and safety criteria and some form of quality control (QC) for components. Surface systems can be located indoors and outdoors, be natural or artificial (or a combination), and thus are subject to a number of influences, including a broad range of functional-related serviceability requirements. An example of a long-pile artificial turf pitch is presented in schematic form in Figure 3.1 showing the general components, with further details on surface construction provided in Chapter 2.

A sports surface, or any construction for any specific sport, is in general required to adhere to all or most of the following general principles (modified from BS 7044 Part 1, 1990):

- It should be identifiable in objective terms and be differentiated from other products on the basis of suitable descriptors including physical and performance-related factors.
- It should be comprised of components that are consistent in composition and quality, ideally to an agreed certified standard.
- It should be capable of being maintained after installation to provide consistent playing performance for an appropriate period of time/use.
- It should provide appropriate properties such that the user to surface interaction can be conducted safely, while the user can perform sporting skills to an appropriate level. For most sports this interaction is through the shoe–surface contact while running, turning and jumping/landing etc. It should provide some safety-related properties for falls and sliding if appropriate to the sport, and for interaction of users' equipment (e.g. hockey sticks).
- It should provide, for ball-related sports, appropriate ball to surface interaction for bounce, roll and spin.
- It should provide appropriate resistance to general degradation of the surface integrity through use and the environment, or accidental damage from water, chemical attack or fire, for general user/public safety (indoors or outdoors).
- It should have a suitable expected life for the proposed use.
- It should, ideally if planned, provide appropriate stable interactions for non-specific use by the general public at spectator or non-sporting events.

The above list could be updated to include more modern concerns such as:

- It should not cause any adverse effect on the local environment through materials contained within it and released during degradation processes.
- It should ideally contain materials that are recyclable or re-usable at the end of life, to an appropriate extent.

Having defined these key principles, it is clear that to achieve these many functions the surfaces must have a large range of suitable properties or facets of behaviour. These properties clearly include material properties related to both player–surface and ball–surface interactions. In addition the surface should be resilient to wear and comprised of safe elements/chemicals. These properties and attributes may need to be tested for the separate material components, stages of manufacture and installation, and in-service as a complete 'system' at initial life and later life.

### *Why are surfaces tested?*

In general, for the measurement and assessment of sports surface systems, commercial organisations exist that supply specialist testing services and advice. These companies are themselves subject to quality assurance standards for accreditation and audited periodically. Some sports governing bodies also require a further periodic gathering of these 'test institutes' to demonstrate the operators' test methods and apparatus efficacy.

The rationale for testing sports surface systems includes the following key objectives:

- To compare surface systems – for cost and quality.
- To provide comparison to a 'standard' – for components and/or systems (e.g. for products and installations).
- To monitor in-service performance, support decision-making regarding maintenance process requirements and/or accreditation for competitive sports use.
- To investigate material/system properties for research – assisting product development, testing ideas, evaluating behaviour and linking to 'performance' for safety or skill – and developing new test methods.

To meet the testing objectives, a range of tests and test methods have been developed and implemented over many years, and new test methods do appear and disappear with experience. However, as surfaces become more sophisticated and the science of user–surface interaction is progressed, it is apparent that there is scope to add to the suite of tests already used in practice and to better critically appraise many of the traditional tests for their suitability and develop or modify these through research. A discussion of the possible future directions for sports surface testing is set out at the end of this chapter.

## Overview of testing standards and their development (UK focus)

A 'standard' is a published document that contains a technical specification or other precise criteria designed to be used consistently as a rule, guideline or definition. Standards help to make life simpler when comparing products and increase the reliability and the effectiveness of many goods and services. They represent a summary of best practice and are created by bringing together the experience and expertise of all interested parties – the producers, sellers, buyers, users and regulators of a particular material, product, process or service.

There is now a very large set of sports-surface-related standards and associated sport-specific test requirements and performance-related acceptability limits, too many to fully describe in a book chapter and hence only the key ones are included here.

In Europe, the process to harmonise the national standards from each member country is essentially complete for sports surfaces, and these standards are subsequently reviewed approximately every five years by technical committees in each country and proposed changes voted upon. The test methods and guidance are, however, continually evolving – specifically it is observed in relation to developments and challenges raised by the widening acceptance of artificial turf at elite (professional) level. In addition, new standards emerge as experience grows with newer apparatus, for which a recent example is the Advanced Artificial Athlete mechanical test which combines the features of the previous Berlin Artificial Athlete and the Stuttgart Athlete apparatus, with some new features to measure a value for 'energy recovery'. The test method is not yet an approved European standard, but exists in current IGB performance standards, explained further in the section 'Player–surface test methods' later in this chapter. In addition, the performance limits set by NGB/IGBs continue to evolve as greater experience is developed, for which a recent example is an increase in minimum drop height relating to the 'Head Injury Criterion' test in World Rugby (WR) guidance, also further detailed in the section 'Player–surface test methods'.

Elsewhere in the world, standards organisations such as the American Society for Testing Materials (ASTM), and the International Organisation for Standards (ISO) have similar updating procedures to those in Europe. It is of note, however, that the three key international sports governing bodies (hockey – FIH, soccer – FIFA, and Rugby Union – World Rugby) stipulate primarily European test standards.

### *History of standards*

In the UK the original sports-surface-testing British Standard was published in four parts as BS 7044. This included aspects of classification, selection, performance requirements and test methods, and multi-sport use. Part 1 comprising classification and general introduction was last updated and published in 1990. This standard was borne out of the previous guidance stipulated by the 'Sports Council Specification for Artificial Sport Surfaces' (Sports Council, 1984), which was 'developed in collaboration and cooperation of the equipment manufacturers and governing bodies of sport to standardise test methods, to specify requirements for durability, playing performance and safety and to give guidance on the characteristics of artificial surfaces'. BS 7044 was primarily intended 'to be of interest to local and education authorities, universities, schools and sports clubs to guide them when purchasing a sports surface'. The performance requirements given in BS 7044 reflect mainly 'the needs of recreational, educational and clubs but may also be satisfactory for top level competition'. The collaborating bodies that were represented included the Sports Turf Research Institute (STRI), the Rubber and Plastics Research Association Technology Ltd (RAPRA), the Building Research Establishment, and Textiles Institute, among many more. Many of these organisations had already introduced testing standards in their own fields of application, and the diversity of information led to the need for a common set of standards for sports surfaces.

Prior to this important standard a comprehensive publication by Graham Tipp and Vic Watson, then working for the Greater London Council (Tipp and Watson, 1982), titled *Polymeric Surfaces for Sport and Recreation*, was perhaps the first useful reference on many aspects of sports surfaces. The book, 400 pages long, covers many aspects and facets of surface materials, requirements and behaviour, aimed at educating technologists and users/specifiers. It deals with applications, material characteristics and methods of manufacture and installation, degradation, maintenance, and user-focused assessment and monitoring techniques. The authors included much of their own experience and research findings and opinions, and indeed many of the test methods described therein, still in use today, were of their own development. They went on to found an independent sports surface test house. Graham Tipp was also the first chairman of the British Standards working committee (PRI/57) that both dealt with the introduction of the standards into the UK and initiated the harmonisation of European Standards, many of which were first published circa 2005.

## Key current standards

### *Introduction*

The key European standards are discussed below, superseding the previous British Standards almost in their entirety. However, there is currently no provision of a suitable overview that includes a useful introduction to the topic area, a glossary of useful terms and general advice to help find information most relevant to a specific user – such as that which existed in BS 7044. It is hoped that this can be addressed in the coming years.

The following sub-sections provide an overview of the European standards that cover outdoor and indoor sports facilities. These are in reality 'specifications' and in essence set out the requirements for selection and approval of products and systems. The specifications refer to a lengthy list of further standards for specific test methods and reporting the results, some of which are covered in later sections of this chapter.

### *Outdoor facilities*

Outdoor facilities are comprised of several standards covering sport or product types, with artificial turf fields dealt with separately such that there exist three separate standards as detailed below.

- EN 14877 (2013): Synthetic surfaces for outdoor sports areas – Specification.

This standard specifies the requirements for synthetic surfaces (either placed in situ or prefabricated) for outdoor sports facilities. Its scope covers synthetic surfaces for the following applications: athletics – track and field; tennis; and multi-sports. It is noted that multi-sports means facilities where more than one sport is played on the surface and this may be defined in national documents such that the definition can vary between countries in Europe.

This standard refers to a further 10 EN standards to directly support its application (termed normative references) and these primarily comprise detailed test methods for performance or durability for example. The document specifies 'Requirements for Safety in Use', comprising both the test methods and the compliance limits (e.g. ball rebound height limits for tennis). It specifies 'Material Characteristics', such as resistance to wear, thickness and tensile properties. It also specifies a method for measuring surface regularity, e.g. maximum of 6mm under a 3m straight edge (note: this test method is taken from highways and airfield testing standards). The surfaces may be impermeable or permeable, such that specific drainage design may be required, and minimum water infiltration rates are specified to ensure the surface is again useable soon after rainfall events.

The multi-sports surface systems identified comprise 'hard' surfaces, such as asphalt or concrete. Synthetic turf is dealt with in two separate standards, notwithstanding its use in tennis-specific facilities, as detailed in the next sub-sections.

- EN 15330 'Surfaces for sports areas – Synthetic turf and needle punched surfaces primarily designed for outdoor use'.

This standard comprises two parts. The requirements are intended to apply to surfaces used for community, educational and recreational sport. For professional and elite levels of competition, most sports governing bodies have published their own specifications; the requirements of the sports' governing bodies may differ from those detailed in this European Standard and facility developers are advised to ensure that they select surfaces offering the correct levels of performance for the levels of competition to be played on the pitch or court. This European Standard is based on type approval testing of products in the laboratory. Selected requirements may also be used on-site to assess the suitability of installed surfaces. Guidance on the testing of installations is given in this standard.

- EN 15330 Part 1 (2013): Specification for synthetic turf.

This specifies requirements for (primarily) outdoor surfaces comprised of synthetic turf for performance and durability for sports including hockey, association football, rugby union, tennis and multi-sports use. The requirements set out are aimed at surfaces for community, educational and recreational use. The document refers to a further 31 EN and ISO standards, detailed test methods, and includes use of generic test methods from other industries and applications, for example for aggregates, textile floor coverings and general plastics and rubber (e.g. hardness) testing (ISO standards). Synthetic turf is defined as 'a sports surface comprised of a carpet of tufted, knitted or woven construction whose pile is designed to replicate the appearance of natural grass'.

The 'general requirements' section specifies several tests and compliance limits for assessing resistance to artificial weathering: colour fastness; tensile strength of the yarn; water infiltration rate, strength of synthetic turf carpet joints and abrasion resistance. It specifies the test methods and compliance limits for specific sports applications and multi-sports applications. Within each sport category the test methods are aimed to specify both ball behaviour and player interaction tests. In addition, a mechanical wear test is specified which comprises applying cycles of a loaded roller to simulate footwear abrasion. The test positions for field assessment of complete installations are specified, and these are different for the sport categories. The annexes also stipulate related information and standards, such as that information regarding maintenance should be supplied by the manufacturer/contractor, limits for surface regularity and a detailed list for product identification – which refers to a further list of 12 EN and ISO test standards, for example particle size of infill materials, pile fibre identification by calorimetry method, and a categorisation approach for synthetic carpet products based on pile length, carpet mass per unit area and tuft withdrawal force.

- EN 15330 Part 2 (2008), details the 'Specification for needle-punched surfaces'.

This is very similar to, and complements, Part 1 and is aimed at the more specialist and niche market for the method of manufacture of synthetic turf by needle punching and is aimed at those products for either multi-sport use or tennis-specific use. In principle it contains the same requirements and general contents as Part 1, and as such is not dealt with further here.

### *Indoor facilities*

Indoor floors may be comprised of many components, both artificial and natural (e.g. wood). Additional requirements are included in the standards relating to indoor facilities for health and safety reasons, primarily for fire and smoke risk to occupants and visibility (which can include lighting standards – not included here).

- EN 14904 (2006): Surfaces for sports areas – Indoor surfaces for multi-sports use – Specification.

This standard covers multi-sport indoor facilities, excluding indoor tennis halls, and includes general use for physical education. It includes requirements for products, test methods and evaluation of conformity. It refers to a further 18 EN or ISO standards, essential to its application. Many of the normative references are primarily detailed test methods, and these include aspects of fire risk and classification, coatings such as paints and varnishes (e.g. measurement of specular gloss, abrasion resistance) and formaldehyde release in wood-based panels.

The standard classifies floors by their expected general response to load as either area elastic, point elastic, combined elastic or mixed-elastic, as detailed in Chapter 2 (see Figure 3.2 and also the next section).

The general requirements regarding safety of the user are set out, primarily comprising test methods for impact (shock-absorption) and vertical deformation under load. It is noted that temperature may affect the properties and performance, and applied strain rates, for testing. Surface slip resistance (friction) is also specified. In addition to the player and ball performance-related tests, resistance of the floor to damage from rolled-out spectator seating is a requirement, plus level of indentation and repeated impact limits to protect against damage.

There is a large amount of detail in this standard regarding requirements to meet legislation for construction products. For example, fire-resistance rating and measurement of formaldehyde emissions are requirements. The flooring components must comply with 'conformity' requirements, primarily through a documented factory production control procedure (FPC). The FPC is a quality assurance process that includes a system for checking the control of raw materials, the process control, calibration plan, finished product testing and traceability. It states,

> Many products come under European Directives, and to be placed on the market in the European Union, some must bear CE marking

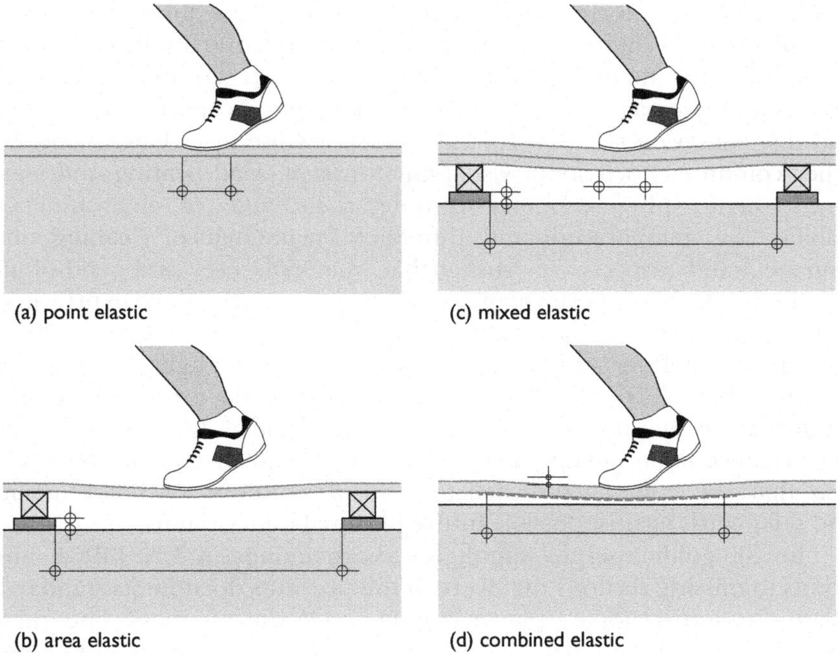


*Figure 3.2* Indoor floor categorisation based upon structure and behaviour under load showing the four classes: (a) point elastic; (b) area elastic; (c) mixed elastic; and (d) combined elastic (reproduced with permission from Sport England, 2007).

– a legal requirement. CE marking is the manufacturer's claim that the product meets the essential requirements of all relevant European Directives.

If a manufacturer claims their product complies and it does not, they can be prosecuted.

- Floors for Indoor Sports – Design Guidance Note (Sport England, 2007).

In the UK Sport England published their indoor floor design guidance in 1999 and updated it in September 2007 to reflect the publication of the European standard 14904. This guidance note is aimed at users, specifiers and clients (facility owner/operators).

This guidance document is different to the European standards in that it both explains what is in the standards regarding tests and limits and, to an extent, explains why these are relevant and raises issues surrounding the shortcomings or limitations of the standards.

The document discusses the range of floors available for indoor sports. It explains the requirements for different sports, and multi-sport, with implications for the design, cost and construction. It sets out in simple-to-understand language the key issues for selection of a sports floor system, and discusses aspects of: sports use; non-sports use (e.g. dance, concerts, other community activities); visual environment; load bearing and wear requirements; physical injury considerations; role of environmental stability (i.e. temperature and humidity); maintenance, cleaning and hygiene; and aspects of sustainable material use and end-of-life considerations. Sport performance requirements are explained in principle, explaining the need for measuring specific characteristics of the floor behaviour for player and ball interaction. The Sport England (SE) guide explains the role of the European standard 14904, within its section 'Performance Standards'. The role of the detailed test methods and performance limits is emphasised to ensure compliance of products and also that the completed installation ensures aspects of build quality and safeguards against possible future personal injury claims.

The SE guide usefully highlights shortcomings in EN 14904, and points to missing sections that were in the previous documents/standards relating to impact forces, player fatigue and surface flatness. The guide also includes a very informative section on construction aspects of indoor floors, covering the materials used and their desirable properties and limitations, the role of the sub-floor support system and damp proofing, surface treatments and underfloor heating. A further section explains the considerations needed for equipment and their fixings, and colour and court markings. The document's appendices include a summary of the floor types and the force reduction and vertical deformation limits; guidance for multi-sport floors and compatibility between specific sport requirements and EN 14904; and guidance for specialist facilities (e.g. indoor running tracks).

Multi-use facilities, also termed multi-use games areas (MUGAs),

> offer a cost-effective solution for schools and other facilities with a wide range of sporting demands. While a multi-sports area is often seen as a 'safe option', it should be recognised that there will almost always be a need for compromise, primarily in terms of the performance of the playing surface, as no one surface is suitable for all types of sport.
>
> (EN 15330)

Furthermore, the compromise on the player/surface interactions is considered more difficult if players are to be protected from an increased risk of injury. For example, reducing the shock-absorption level to increase the ball rebound for tennis (i.e. harder surface) might result in a greater number of injuries to football players who will fall onto the surface more frequently than tennis players. It is suggested that, as a general rule, the characteristics of the surface should be designed to satisfy the priority sports for the facility.

## Overview of international governing body requirements (European elite sport focus)

For the elite sporting level of competition, specific guidelines for artificial surfaces for athletics and synthetic turf for hockey have been in existence for many years. The IGBs published handbooks of requirements to ensure that for international and Olympic-level competitions (e.g. athletics: IAAF, 2008; tennis: ITF, 2012; hockey: FIH, 2014) appropriate consistency was achieved in the performance of the surfaces utilised, albeit within an acceptable range of values. In more recent times these handbooks have become more detailed, largely due to association football (FIFA, 2012a) and rugby union (World Rugby, 2012) introducing their own standards for artificial turf systems, and the number of test methods stipulated therein has multiplied to implement experience and attempt to better replicate the properties of natural turf. Rugby League is a more recent addition to the IGB list with artificial turf guidance now in their facilities information and rules (RFL, 2011), and their guide is very closely aligned to that of World Rugby. The IGB handbooks are generally available to download for free from their websites, in addition to related useful information about specific rules and player welfare.

In the case of tennis the increasing speed of the game through player conditioning, racquet technology and newer surface technologies, has led to more regulation and more test methods – though these are not all published standards. The ITF Technical Commission is responsible for monitoring developments in equipment technology in order to protect the nature of the game of tennis at all levels. As custodians of the Rules of Tennis, the ITF has the sometimes difficult task of judging whether innovations in tennis equipment may bring about a benefit to those who play, or whether such developments constitute a threat to the nature of the game (ITF, 2012).

The IAAF is responsible for issuing certificates for athletics facilities that meet their requirements (IAAF, 2008), for levels of competition termed Class 1 or 2. These certificates are valid until either the track or field is resurfaced or repairs are carried out, or the surface is re-marked. Track products are classed as certified products if they meet the requirements, and registered as such for a period of four years.

Since the late 1990s, the outdoor team sports of association soccer, rugby union and more recently rugby league have gradually evolved their guidelines to manage the introduction of artificial turf into the laws of the game, with a view to protect the players' safety and maintain the levels of play performance akin to natural turf. The levels of play performance stipulated are, however, different for different levels of competition and for community use. In all of these sports' requirements the acceptable values for compliance of the play performance tests comprise a range of values, for example ball rebound may be stipulated as between 0.6 and 1.0 metre in association football to comply with the FIFA 1-star rating (community level). As a result there exists variation in the way any one pitch type is permitted to vary from another, and it then may vary in performance through its lifetime and still comply with the stipulated requirements. In most instances it is apparent the sport governing bodies have been through a period of research, testing and monitoring of facilities, qualitatively and quantitatively, to develop and update their play performance requirements.

In general the play performance limits relate to a series of laboratory and/or field tests to measure aspects of ball-to-surface and player-to-surface interaction. In addition tests are required to verify product identification, manufacturing quality and durability. The governing bodies have also developed either recommendations or stipulated requirements for the 'approval' of artificial sports surface products to be used in their sport such that manufacturers may show that their products comply with the IGB requirements and use this in their product marketing. Thus, there are aspects of approval of manufactured products based on laboratory testing, and also for approval of installations through field testing. The formal approval of a product to an international governing body (IGB) standard stipulates that the compliance testing is carried out by an approved sport-specific 'Test Institute' and these specialist companies have to demonstrate regularly that their equipment and procedures meet the highest standards of best practice (e.g. ISO 17025 which covers quality assurance of testing services). The IGBs publish, on their websites, lists of approved products and installations and also the approved Test Institutes. There are several such Test Institutes in Europe, and currently three in the UK.

The framework for approval of products and facilities is now often termed the 'quality concept' (QC) or similar. This approval framework is explained in the next section, and the information presented has a bias toward association football whereby the IGB (FIFA) have, it appears, invested a lot of resources into developing very fulsome guidance for artificial turf's introduction at both the elite and community levels.

## *'Quality concept' for testing and approval of sports surfaces*

There exists a similar methodology for performance compliance assessment and approval of sports surface products and newly installed systems, usually comprising the following steps for approval:

1 Accreditation of a manufacturer's products for use in the specific sport – based on the complete surface 'system' (i.e. carpet, infill and shockpad for example) achieving the limits set for compliance stated in the performance standard for the sport (or cross-referenced to the EN specifications as discussed previously). This allows the product vendor to show that their surface system has been approved by that sport for a specific level of play performance for competition, or community level and/or multi-sport use.
2 Accreditation of a constructed system – based upon the finished installed system passing a series of field tests required to meet the compliance targets. This is similar to the laboratory suite of tests in 1, above, focused on play performance tests related to the users and balls, but usually also includes build quality (e.g. seams, planarity, uniformity, drainage and so on). There usually exists more than one level of performance rating for a facility, related to the level of competition. For example in hockey international and national levels differ slightly and for football a 1-star and 2-star scheme exists for community and professional levels respectively. The field 'certification' testing usually occurs within a few months of construction completion, often not immediately to allow the system to 'bed in' through some use and the initial maintenance programme.
3 Long-term performance – based upon retesting the system at intervals, often the same or similar to the testing suite described in 2, above, to demonstrate ongoing quality at the specific level the facility was originally designed for. The frequency of re-testing is dictated by the competition play level 'rating' of the system (e.g. for FIFA 1 or 2 star approval in their 'quality concept') and may be every two years for example for World Rugby and one year for FIFA 2 star.

The 'Quality Concept for Football Turf' (FQC) developed by FIFA for artificial turf is explained further here as a good example (FIFA, 2012a). The FQC was introduced in 2001, and was at the time a more rigorous test programme for artificial turf than had previously existed. Note FIFA favour the alternative term 'football turf' rather than artificial turf. The FQC was put in place to assess the ball–surface interaction, player–surface interaction and durability of products to allow successful manufacturers to enter into a licensing programme to use the prestigious 'FIFA Recommended' logo. In 2004 FIFA introduced artificial surfaces into the Laws of the Game, and their FQC was further developed to introduce two categories of performance. The two-star rating was aimed at professional competition and training to replicate the playing qualities of the best-quality natural turf pitches – based on their research and field testing of turf pitches. The one-star rating was aimed at facilities for training and community use, and lower-level competition, and sets slightly wider bands of acceptability limits for the test results but a more intensive requirement for the likely higher usage of the facility.

The FIFA guidance is fulsome, including two separate booklets, the first titled the 'FIFA Quality Concept for Football Turf, Handbook of Requirements' (FIFA 2012a) which sets out the rigorous programme of compliance that is required, including limits for acceptability for product compliance and play performance compliance. A related handbook is titled 'FIFA Quality Concept for Football Turf, Handbook of Test Methods' (FIFA, 2012b) and details the specifics of the test apparatus and procedures to be followed. The FIFA manuals refer to a number of EN and ISO standards, and also include modifications to the published standards to suit their own requirements. The handbook of tests is aimed at artificial turf but the tests can be used to assess the relative performance of natural turf. A key principle in the testing philosophy adopted is that the 'tests shall be made on all elements of the construction that influence the sports performance or biomechanical response of the surface' (FIFA, 2012b). In practice, much of the surface system testing in the laboratory is done on a 'rigid' concrete floor to simulate the rigidity of a bound base in the field. However, if the field is to be constructed onto stone (termed a 'dynamic' base), which may contribute to the dynamic performance of the surface, then a similar base is required to be constructed in the laboratory. The FIFA testing handbook is very prescriptive, stipulating sample sizes, preparation requirements (for example including conditioning of systems by rolling with a studded roller), wetting procedures, temperature control and others. The test methods detailed comprise a helpful explanation of the test principle, the apparatus required, the test procedure and also the calculation and expression of results.

In brief summary (also detailed with other sports in Tables 3.1 and 3.2), the FIFA ball–surface tests comprise: vertical ball rebound; angled ball rebound (using a ball launch cannon); and ball roll distance from an inclined ramp. The FIFA player–surface tests comprise three measures from the same fixed energy dynamic impact apparatus: the shock absorption (hardness); surface vertical deformation; and energy restitution; and for friction/traction it comprises: rotational resistance (grip); linear friction (grip); and a (indirect) measure of skin/surface friction.

The FIFA durability laboratory tests comprise, in brief: simulated mechanical abrasion using repeated cycles of two studded rollers; and artificial weathering. Performance tests are done before and after abrasion to assess durability performance, and after the artificial weathering to assess the effects on colour, and fibre tensile strength. Assessment of the synthetic infill is required, for example to determine the particle size, and of the ratio of organic to inorganic material present.

The key performance-related test methods and apparatus are explained in further detail later in this chapter.

The FIFA Quality Concept is aimed at the certification of a particular football field that has been found to fully meet all the requirements. FIFA did not intend it as a simple product approval system. A FIFA 'licensee' needs to undertake the laboratory and field testing, and operate a programme of factory quality control (set out in their requirements handbook, FIFA 2012b). Once certified, a field must then be re-tested periodically to maintain the FIFA certification. Currently the period is 12 months for a FIFA two-star approved facility.

In more recent years, World Rugby has launched a very similar scheme to that of FIFA's termed 'Regulation 22' (World Rugby, 2012). Rugby union has sport-specific concerns over player injury that led to the introduction of several extra tests with regard to surface hardness for possible head injury, and it increased some aspects of surface durability requirements for resistance to damage from the heavier players, longer studs and the effects of rugby-specific play such as scrummaging and rucking. World Rugby included a caveat in Regulation 22 regarding liability for any loss or injury to be carried by the pitch manufacturer/installer for artificial products to protect World Rugby from any claims. In addition, the installer, or the regional union, have to carry a minimum of £5 million pubic liability insurance to cover against injury claims through participation in rugby matches. World Rugby have a proactive scheme for recording injuries on artificial turf to assist them in their aim to evaluate the ongoing safety of artificial turf in comparison to natural turf. FIFA have also carried out similar research, which is available on its website.

A flow diagram describing the steps in approving a new sports surface facility is shown in Figure 3.3. In addition to the play performance and durability testing, it should be noted that in many instances aspects of construction quality are also verified during the works as part of the quality assurance process and final approvals. The construction testing is often termed 'key stage inspections'.

Table 3.1 presents a brief overview of the general properties that require testing for the major sports' international governing bodies that utilise artificial surfaces, including hockey, athletics and tennis in addition to those detailed previously.

Other sports bodies do have a different approach to that of football and rugby however. Tennis, for example, is different in that its test requirements and specified court properties are specifically aimed at ball–surface behaviour, not player–surface interaction. No details of any requirements for player–surface behaviour are in existence, though this is considered likely to change to include some measure of court grip/friction. The ITF has a specific system to classify court speed or 'pace' of the ball after impact, which can be used to select an appropriate surface

*Table 3.1* Summary overview of common IGB performance-related testing requirements.

| *Property* | | *Sport (international governing body)* | | | | | |
|---|---|---|---|---|---|---|---|
| | | *Association Football (FIFA)* | *Rugby Union (World Rugby)* | *Rugby League (RFL)* | *Field Hockey (FIH)* | *Athletics (IAAF)* | *Tennis (ITF)* |
| Player surface | Shock absorption | Y | Y | Y | Y | Y | N |
| | Energy restitution | N | Y | Y | N | N | N |
| | Deformation | Y | Y | Y | Y | Y | N |
| | Head impact | N | Y | Y | N | N | N |
| | Skin friction/abrasion | Y[1] | Y[1] | Y[1] | N | N | N |
| | Grip/traction | Y | Y | Y | Y | Y | N |
| Ball surface | Vertical rebound height | Y | Y | Y | Y | n/a | Y |
| | Angled rebound/pace | Y[1] | Y[1] | Y[1] | Y[1] | n/a | Y |
| | Roll distance | Y | N | N | Y | n/a | N |
| | Roll deviation | N | N | N | Y | n/a | N |
| Identification testing[1] | Mass per unit area | Y | Y | Y | Y | Y | N |
| | Tufts per unit area | Y | Y | Y | Y | n/a | N |
| | Pile length/surface thickness | Y | Y | Y | Y | Y | N |
| | Pile weight | Y | Y | Y | Y | n/a | N |
| | DCS | Y | Y | Y | Y | n/a | N |
| | Yarn cross-section and thickness | Y | Y | Y | Y | n/a | N |
| | Performance infill classification | Y | Y | Y | Y | n/a | N |
| | Stabilising infill classification | Y | Y | Y | Y | n/a | N |

| Property | | Sport (international governing body) | | | | | |
|---|---|---|---|---|---|---|---|
| | | Association Football (FIFA) | Rugby Union (World Rugby) | Rugby League (RFL) | Field Hockey (FIH) | Athletics (IAAF) | Tennis (ITF) |
| Durability, climatic and material testing[1] | Simulated wear (LISport) | Y | Y | Y | Y | N | N |
| | Wear taber | N | N | N | Y | Y | N |
| | Elevated temperature testing | Y | Y | Y | N | Y | N |
| | Reduced temperature testing | Y | Y | Y | N | Y | N |
| | UV resistance | Y | Y | Y | Y | Y | N |
| | Joint strength | Y | Y | Y | Y | N | N |
| | Tuft withdrawal strength | Y | Y | Y | Y | n/a | N |
| | Porosity | Y | Y | Y | Y | Y | N |
| | Tensile strength | Y | Y | Y | Y | Y | N |
| In-situ measurements | Surface evenness | Y | Y | Y | Y | Y | Y |
| | Slope | N | Y | Y | Y | Y | Y |
| | Planarity | N | N | N | Y | N | Y |
| | Porosity | N | N | N | Y | Y | N |
| | Line dimensions | Y | Y | Y | Y | Y | Y |
| | Infill depth/evenness | Y | Y | Y | Y | n/a | N |
| | Visual inspection | Y | Y | Y | Y | Y | Y |

1 Laboratory testing only

Note: Many other sports and specific regions have their own standards which are commonly based around the test methods above. These include but are not limited to: GAA, ECB, AFL, Nordic Standards, Netball, etc.

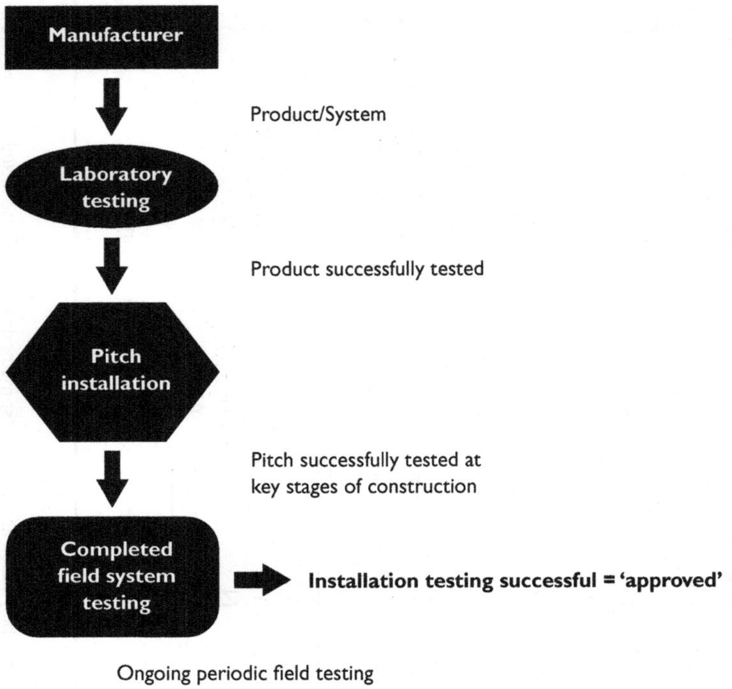


*Figure 3.3* A schematic showing the generic process of achieving approval of a surface system and field installation in accordance with the quality concept schemes typified by the FIFA/World Rugby/RFL and FIH international governing body schemes for artificial turf.

or a ball for that surface (from an approved list of three types of ball). Court pace is classified as either: Category 1 (slow); Category 2 (medium-slow); Category 3 (medium); Category 4 (medium-fast); Category 5 (fast). A product can have an 'approved' classification, and be placed on a list, for three years. Facilities can be approved (for the day of testing) and gain a status for 'quality of installation'. However, apart from the major tennis tournaments court testing is not mandatory.

The ITF has identified 'definitive' and 'predictive' methods for testing the key properties of a surface. Definitive methods are recommended for laboratory testing and on-site testing of courts for professional competition. Predictive methods provide a more economical means of on-site testing. ITF recognition is an acknowledgement that a court meets the recommendations provided in the ITF Guide to Test Methods for Tennis Court Surfaces (ITF, 2012). ITF recognition is targeted at venues hosting elite-level competitions where the standard of play demands the specification of precise playing characteristics, e.g. at international tournaments and national/regional tennis centres. There are two levels of

ITF recognition (ITF recognition is not mandatory, nor does it imply any form of ITF approval or endorsement):

- One-star ITF recognition – the court is tested for quality of installation.
- Two-star ITF recognition – in addition to the one-star tests, the court is tested for pace.

ITF recognition is retained until the court is resurfaced or for ten years, whichever is the sooner. However, the results are only valid for the day of testing. Properties of the court may change due to factors such as ambient conditions, use and maintenance.

It is interesting to note that whilst the IGBs have produced much guidance on artificial turf there is little specific guidance relevant to natural turf performance. This situation is expected to change, however, as the sporting bodies are currently researching natural turf in more detail, perhaps due to increasing concern in general over natural turf durability and pressures on professional sports clubs to maximise their assets – in many cases the competition pitch is a key asset. In the case of rugby union there are some useful guidelines for natural turf quality on the World Rugby website. This guidance suggests a set of performance criteria and targets for natural turf to meet a national playing standard, comprising hardness and traction. Hardness is specified from testing with a light Clegg hammer (mass 0.5kg) and it states preferred limits of 50–100g. For (rotational) traction (EN 15301-1) it states preferred limits of >35Nm with 15mm long football studs (World Rugby, 2013). No other tests are specified though it is advised that surface evenness and stud penetration may be useful further assessments. It appears that these guidelines and test methods are aimed at the facility ground staff to maintain appropriate performance levels.

### *Approach to field testing – positions and other factors*

World Rugby states that 'when a field is tested it must satisfy the requirements of all the testing specified in any position on the field'. However locations are specified in its handbook and it further suggests test positions should avoid seams or inlaid lines and that no maintenance activities should occur during testing. Suggested acceptable temperature and wind ranges are specified to avoid undue bias of results. Visual assessment of a field is also incorporated to avoid obvious defects that spot testing may not readily identify, such as any damaged, loose or protruding furniture/carpet (sockets, bungs, yarn or seams etc.). In addition, more recent changes to World Rugby and FIFA guidelines increased the number of test positions for specific tests, such as surface shock-absorption, from 6 to 19.

A sample of the governing bodies' test location information is shown in Figure 3.4.

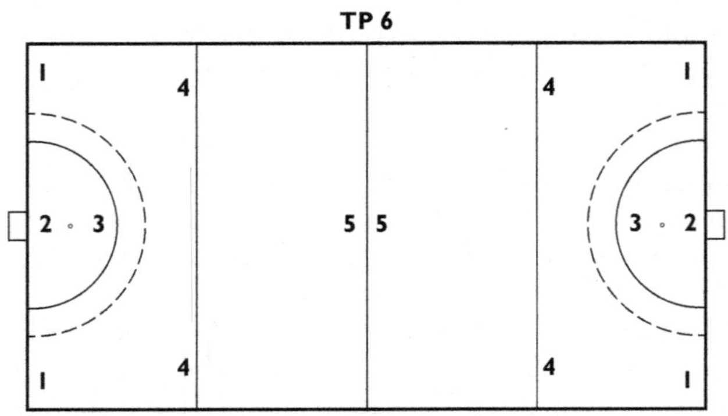


(a) FIH, Field Hockey (note position 6 is in the run off area)

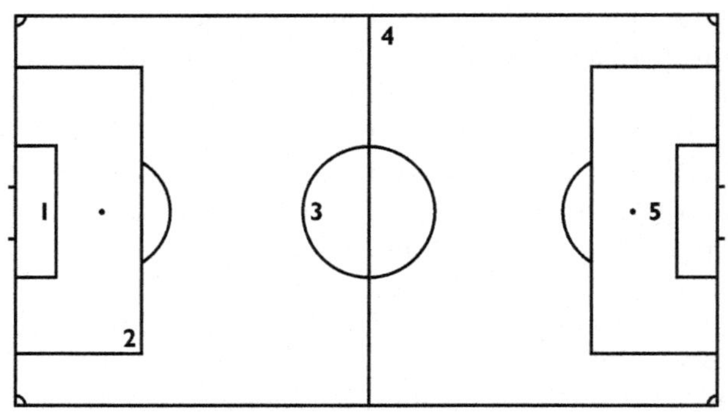


(b) EN 15330, e.g. Association Football or multi-sport use

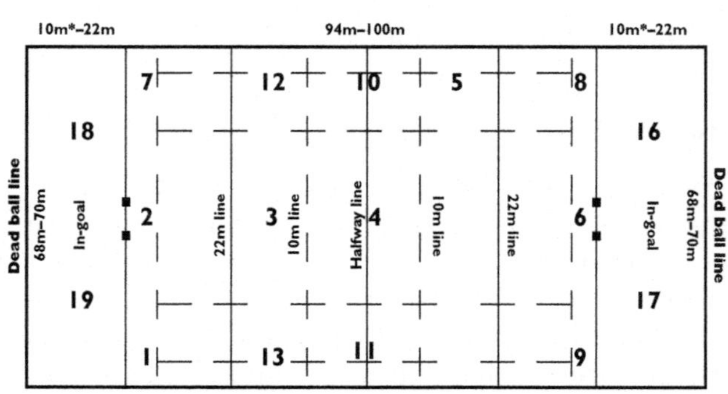


(c) World Rugby, rugby union field

*Figure 3.4* Spot-test locations recommended for field evaluation testing of sports surface systems for: (a) field hockey spot-test positions* (FIH, 2014); (b) EN 15330 general positions (e.g. association football), typical test positions to reflect cross-field wear (6); and (c) World Rugby, rugby union – 19 positions. Note FIFA also require 19 positions for specific tests (FIFA, 2012).

## Maintenance and surface testing

### *Introduction*

All sports surface systems require, or benefit from, some form of maintenance. This is increasingly recognised in the information given in handbooks by all the sports governing bodies and also the industry in general, e.g. through codes of practice (SAPCA, 2009). Prior to the more widespread introduction of artificial turf into many outdoor sports in the 1990s, it may be fair to suggest that once installed the surface maintenance was not always high on the agenda of the owner/operator, and many artificial surface products were perhaps sold into the market as 'all weather' and 'low-maintenance'. The different surface types have different needs, as explained in Chapter 2, but all have a basic need for removal of loose detritus and cleaning if any extraneous products build up that may affect underfoot friction and angled ball bounce, or aesthetics and line markings. The subject of maintenance is not dealt with in great depth here, but the sections below are included as a brief overview and point to some relatively recent research into improving longevity of facilities. Reference is made where applicable to how surfaces degrade and to some useful test methods to characterise degradation of surfaces and changes in performance.

### *Outdoor artificial turf pitches*

Maintenance of artificial turf surfaces has been the topic of much discussion within the industry in recent years (e.g. James and McLeod, 2010). However, the current industry guidance is clearly experience based and anecdotal (Fleming, 2011a). Controlled experimental studies into the effectiveness of maintenance and development of better understanding of the factors affecting the decline in performance of artificial turf systems are currently few and far between in the available literature (McLeod, 2008). There exists little specific guidance from the yarn or carpet manufacturers. Research into maintenance practice and effectiveness would enhance both sports surface science as a whole and lead to test methods more suited to regular monitoring. Ground staff and match referees would benefit from quick, effective assessment of a surface's safety for example.

The maintenance equipment used and specified is often similar to that used in other industry applications such as sweeping and brushing. New maintenance equipment has been developed and patented by some commercial organisations, such as that for deep cleaning long-pile artificial turf fields. However, the claims for effectiveness are arguably not yet substantiated with quantified evidence. There are some within the industry who have argued in the past that too much maintenance may exacerbate wear. Two large studies have advanced understanding of sand-filled carpet systems (McLeod, 2008) and the newer rubber-filled long pile systems (McLaren *et al.*, 2012).

## *Research findings*

The cost and benefit balance between effective maintenance and an outdoor sports surface's longevity, while maintaining a suitable playing standard, has yet to be fully researched and demonstrated with objective data. However James and McLeod (2010) gave useful insight into the relation between increasing levels of contamination in the infill causing a worsening of play performance properties (e.g. increasing surface hardness and increasing ball roll distance) and reduction in surface water infiltration rate leading to possible ponding. This research developed a bespoke test to measure contamination level, comprising a settling tube to separate out the different densities of material excavated from a small area on the surface. The contamination, finer in size, settled last and gave a clear dark layer on top of the sand infill layer. A simple comparison of the heights of the column constituents permitted an estimate of the percentage of contamination (by volume). The effect of contamination volume on the infiltration rate of the surface system is shown in Figure 3.5 (after McLeod, 2008) and demonstrates a large reduction above 5 per cent by weight and potentially failure of the requirements above 10 per cent by weight.

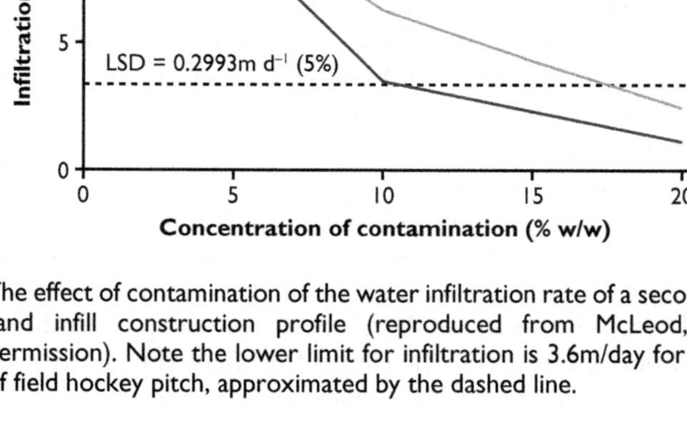


*Figure 3.5* The effect of contamination of the water infiltration rate of a second generation sand infill construction profile (reproduced from McLeod, 2008, with permission). Note the lower limit for infiltration is 3.6m/day for all categories of field hockey pitch, approximated by the dashed line.

The review by McLaren *et al.* (2012) provides a useful discussion of the limited previous research and presents a conceptual model for how a pitch surface may degrade. They reported on one very useful long-term study from Holland (Jan-Kieft, 2009) in which the performance of 50 artificial grass soccer pitches (AGP) built in 2001/02 and retested in 2007 were monitored in relation to FIFA accreditation. Jan-Kieft found that on average these long-pile rubber and sand-filled surfaces became harder and faster, with a higher ball rebound, over time (i.e. usage). The data trend emerged showing that the fields which received higher usage performed the worst and with the greatest change in play performance. Another separate shorter-term study was also reviewed (Joosten *et al.*, 2003), reporting that during the first playing season of six AGPs the ball roll distance had increased on average by a large amount (3.9m) and the surface hardness by a significant amount (force reduction decreased by 5 per cent), which demonstrated a relatively quick change/deterioration in performance. Despite many unknowns in these research studies, the expected trend of a decline in the performance of rubber-filled AGPs with use/time appears to be supported. The specific reasons are perhaps less clear or less clearly evidenced. McLaren *et al.* (2012) developed a useful conceptual model that captures the degradation mechanisms expected to affect the in-service life of an artificial turf pitch. The model was developed from a range of information sources including field research, aspects of material science, and industry experience and observation. The model comprises three elements: the degradation factors, mechanisms and effects (see Figure 3.6). The model has yet to be validated but provides a useful starting point for debate about the complex interaction of the many variables that may effect changes in the surface's performance.

The primary degradation factor highlighted is from the mechanical interaction of players, exacerbated by one or more weathering processes. The introduction of foreign detritus into the AGP system, e.g. fine solids and organic vegetation such as leaves clearly can add to the decline. The mechanisms of degradation describe what happens to the surface components as they are increasingly used and wear ensues. Once one or more of the system effects, which may be measurable, deteriorates to a specific loss of serviceability determined by the testing standards or the users/facility owner, the AGP then reaches the end of its useful life. It is then disposed of, re-used or recycled and replaced with a new system. A strategy for effective maintenance interventions is the goal of the further development of the McLaren model, including appropriate field monitoring. However, it is clear that comprehensive research studies of maintenance effects and benefits require a very large dataset to gather the appropriate evidence.

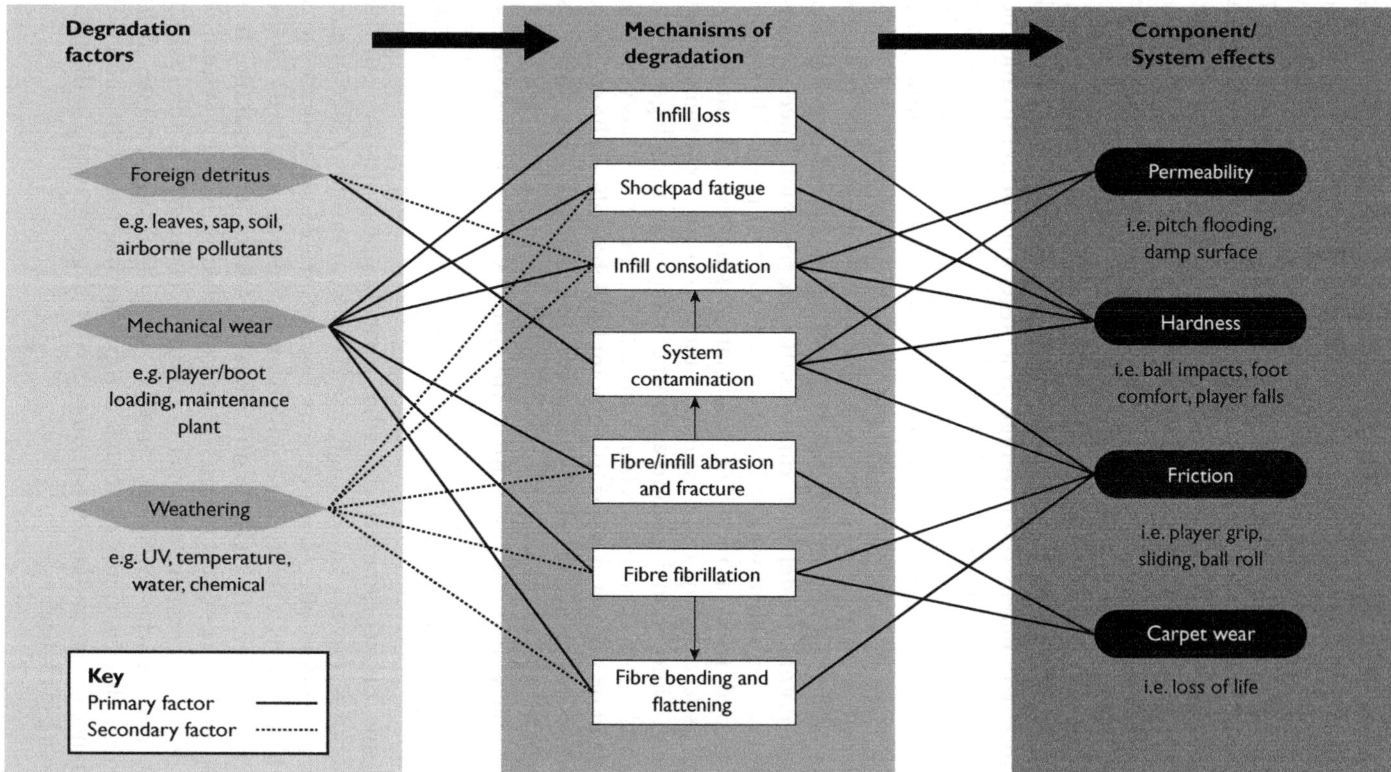


*Figure 3.6* Schematic of a conceptual model for degradation of artificial turf (reproduced from McLaren *et al.* (2012) with permission).

## Performance-related mechanical test methods

### *Introduction*

This section aims to provide some details of several of the key test methods and standards in current use for assessing sports surfaces. The mechanical test methods can in general be classified into groups with similar aims in relation to measuring aspects of player–surface interaction, ball–surface interaction, and material physical properties and durability.

These specific tests are referred to in the relevant European sports surface specifications and in IGB guidance (see earlier sections for an overview of these specific standards and guides). These testing standards are reviewed and can be updated every five years and at the time of writing there are (subtle) changes being made at the relevant European committees. As a consequence the detail in this section may become somewhat outdated and the reader should refer to the most recently published standards. Furthermore, this section aims to provide summary details of key test methods in relation to player- and ball-related testing only, with some comment on their efficacy. Many mechanical tests in existence are necessarily simplistic, and primarily satisfy the objectives of comparing surfaces and providing assurance that they meet specification standards. Many of these industry-standard test methods measure engineering or material properties indirectly, and the results are affected by multiple variables and thus do not provide a strong basis for improving understanding or provide a strong link to the latest research into human movement science or ball physics.

Table 3.2 summarises the target values for approval of surface systems for several key mechanical tests as specified by the IGBs for soccer, rugby, hockey and multi-use facilities. This summary provides a simple comparison across these popular sports and shows the commonality for many of the specified tests. Each of these test methods is detailed further in the subsequent sub-sections.

### *Player–surface test methods*

Player underfoot shock-absorption (hardness) and grip (friction/traction) are generally agreed to be key to movement efficiency and performance, including aspects of injury risk. Skin friction from sliding is a more recent test added initially by FIFA to complement the introduction of softer yarns into longer-pile carpets that supposedly reduced abrasion burns. FIFA recognised the need to assess products in the laboratory for this feature, and the test is quite different to the general friction tests.

*Table 3.2* Summary of performance requirements for synthetic turf

| | *Property* | *Sport (International governing body)* | | | | | | | | | | |
|---|---|---|---|---|---|---|---|---|---|---|---|---|
| | | *Association Football (FIFA)* | | *Rugby Union (World Rugby)* | *Rugby League (RFL)* | | *Field Hockey (FIH)* | | | *EN 15330-1* | | |
| | | *2 star* | *1 star* | | *Stadium* | *Community* | *Global* | *National* | *Multi-sport* | *Football* | *Hockey* | *Multi-sport* |
| Player surface | Shock-absorption (%) | 60–70 | 55–70 | | 50–65 | 50–70 | 40–60 | 40–65 | | 55–70 | ≥ 40 | classification |
| | Energy restitution (%) | – | – | 20–50 | 20–40 | 20–50 | – | – | – | – | – | – |
| | Deformation (mm) | 4–10 | 4–11 | | 3–8.5 | ≤ 11 | – | – | – | 4–10 | 3–10 | – |
| | Head impact criteria (m) | – | – | | ≥ 1.3 | | – | – | – | – | – | – |
| | Rotational resistance (Nm) | 30–45 | 25–50 | | 35–50 | 25–55 | 25–45 | | 25–50 | 25–50 | 25–50 | 25–50 |
| | Slip resistance (–) | – | – | – | – | – | | 0.6–1.0 | | – | – | – |
| | Linear friction-stud deceleration (g) | 3.0–5.5 | 3.0–7.0 | | – | – | – | – | – | – | – | – |
| | Skin friction (μ) | | 0.35–0.75 | | ≤ 0.75 | | – | – | – | – | – | – |
| | Skin abrasion (%) | | | ± 30 | | | – | – | – | – | – | – |
| Ball surface | Vertical rebound height (m or %) | 0.6–0.85 | 0.6–1.0 | | 0.8–1.1 | 0.6–1.1 | 0.1–0.4 | | 0.75–0.4 | 45–75% | ≥ 70% | range |
| | Angled rebound/pace (%) | | 45–80 | | – | – | – | – | – | | – | – |
| | Roll distance (m) | 4–8 | 4–10 | – | – | – | ≥ 10 | ≥ 8 | ≥ 5 | 4–10 | ≥ 8 | range |

Note: EN 15330-1 uses the AA for shock absorption and deformation – all other standards use the AAA; ball rebound for EN 15330-1 is expressed as a percentage. Rotational resistance test foot studs are changed depending on the sport (i.e. different for hockey than football).

*Tests related to impact (vertical)*

The industry measurement standard for (simple) foot surface contact is based on the portable mechanical test device termed the 'Artificial Athlete' (AA, also termed the Berlin Artificial Athlete in some literature) set out in BS EN 14808, 2005. The AA measures the peak impact force from a controlled energy spring-damped impact, from which the parameter 'Force Reduction' is determined, and the same device is adapted by changing the spring (to one of lower stiffness) to measure the surface's vertical deformation under the same impact energy (EN 14809, 2005, also termed the 'Stuttgart test'). The AA test has for a long time represented the 'gold' standard test across many sports, and was originally devised for athletic track testing to represent the 'heel impact' of a heel–toe running action (as shown in Figure 3.7) and measure cushioning behaviour of a surface in simple form. The impact mechanism involves a 20kg mass dropped from 55mm onto a 2000 N/mm helical spring and the impact energy is transferred to the surface through a flat circular bearing plate 70mm in diameter. The load cell records the peak impact force and compares this peak value to a reference force (equation 1) representing a rigid surface, and from these two values the 'force reduction', also termed shock absorbency, value (%) is derived for the surface under test. Three repeat drops are normally done at each test location and the average of the second and third drop reported as the test result.

$$FR = (1 - Fs/Fc) \times 100\ (\%) \qquad \text{Equation 3.1}$$

Where: FR is the force reduction value for the sample in per cent; Fs = the peak force measured on the sample; Fc is the reference peak force for rigid concrete, or a suitable substitute reference value (current guidance stipulates a range between 6350 and 6800N). The per cent force reduction (FR) in general represents the relative hardness of a surface; a larger percentage meaning 'softer' underfoot. A 'hard' surface for tennis for example might produce a FR value of less than 15 per cent.

In 2004 a new test was introduced, the 'Advanced Artificial Athlete' (AAA), which is a modification and amalgamation of the two tests described above. This test is now embedded within the current guidance from FIFA (FIFA, 2012a) and World Rugby (World Rugby, 2012). The AAA uses an accelerometer (in place of the load cell used in the AA), and by manipulation of the impact data records the peak impact force, the peak surface deformation, and the 'energy restitution' for each impact. The energy restitution of a surface, currently expressed as a percentage and derived from the ratio of the rebound velocity to the impact velocity, is currently a topic of debate on whether the surface energy recovery is a factor in player fatigue and how best to measure it.

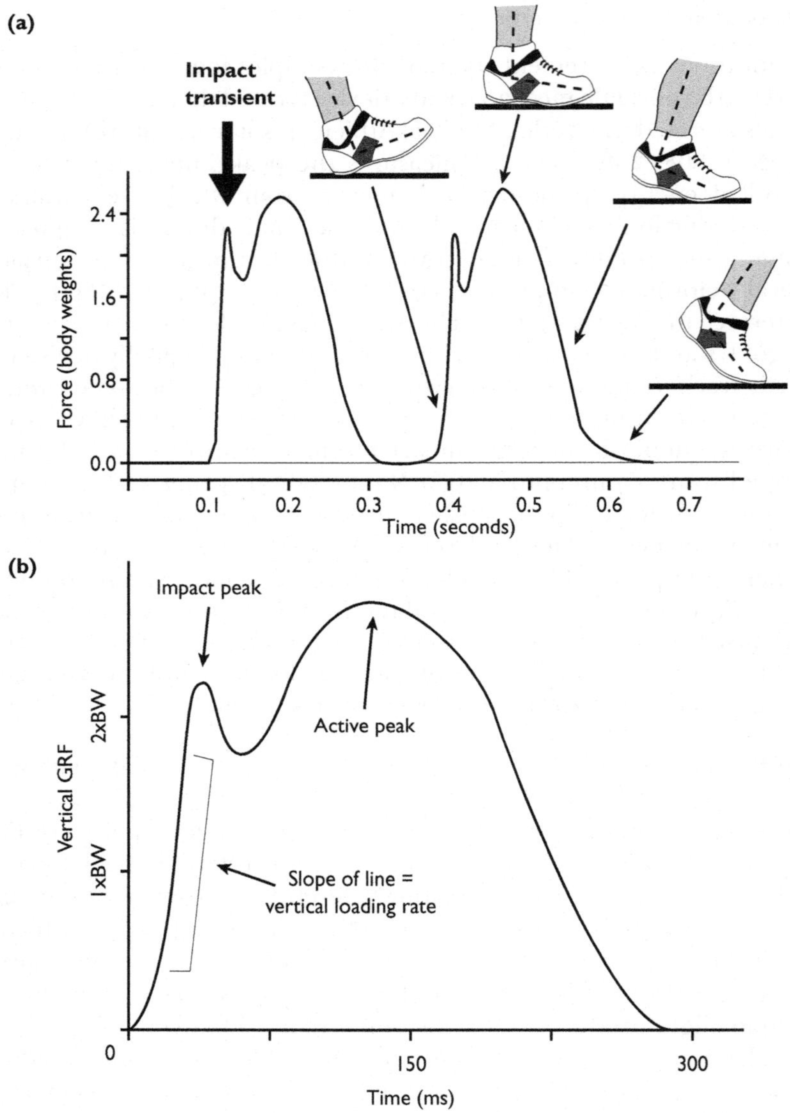


*Figure 3.7* Schematic of: a) heel–toe running action; and b) typical vertical ground reaction forces (GRF) and loading/contact period for each foot contact.

Figure 3.8 shows the AAA device in schematic form, and Figure 3.9 shows the AAA set up on a test sample in the field.

Figure 3.10 shows a graph of force reduction for two short-pile hockey-specific artificial turf carpets (Young, 2006) with a range of thickness of similar shockpad beneath, and demonstrates the large range of force

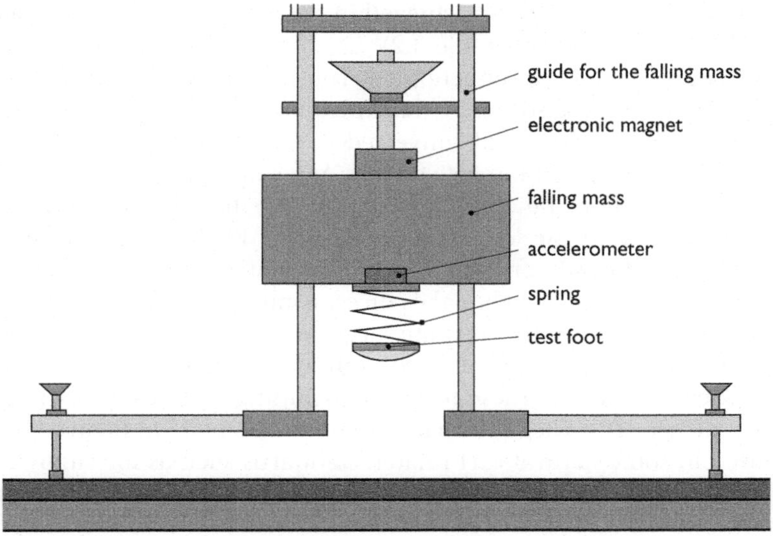


*Figure 3.8* Schematic of the Advaced Artificial Athlete (AAA) device.

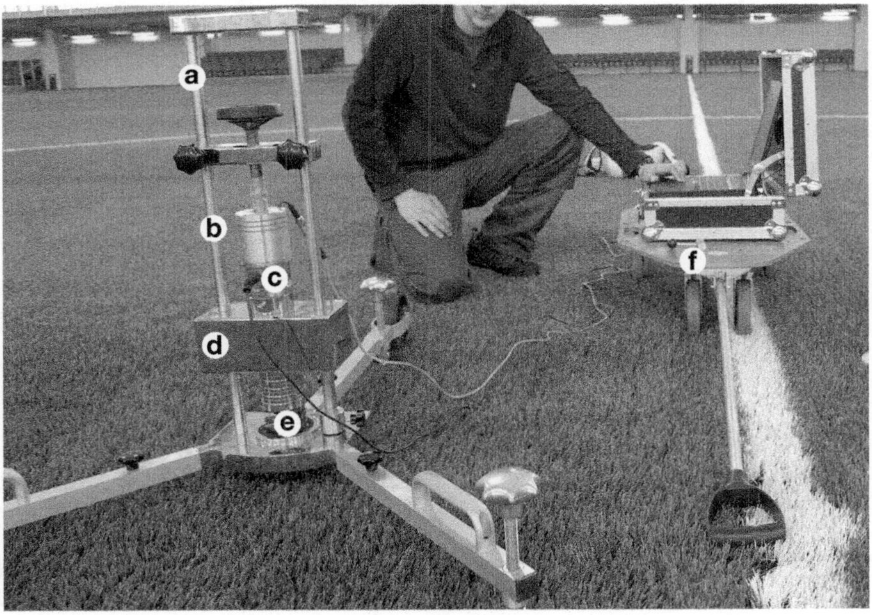


*Figure 3.9* Impact test apparatus, the 'Advanced Artificial Athlete', set up on a long-pile artificial turf field, showing: (a) the guide frame; (b) the release magnet; (c) the load cell; (d) the 20kg drop mass ready to be released; (e) the spring (foot hidden) beneath; and (f) the computer to display the test output results (personal photograph).

reduction values that can be achieved in comparison to the limits set out in the FIH requirements (Table 3.2).

The AA or AAA force reduction (%) is used across a range of sports to rank relative shock-absorbency (hardness) across a range of surfaces. It applies a constant (potential converted to kinetic) energy to the surface under test, at a constant impact velocity. As a consequence, the harder the surface the higher the peak reaction force that is recorded by the accelerometer (and the lower the interpreted FR %). Furthermore, for the AAA the inferred vertical surface deformation is then measured for different peak forces, which makes direct comparison more difficult. The device, although portable, is quite large, relatively heavy to manoeuvre and requires a separate portable computer for data capture and display. In response to some of these features, including cost, a smaller portable impact device, the Clegg Impact Hammer (shown in Figure 3.11) is included in some natural-turf-related standards such as for rugby union (a 0.5kg mass hammer) and non-turf standards for cricket (a 2.25kg mass hammer) (ECB, 2007). It has been used in research studies (Twomey *et*

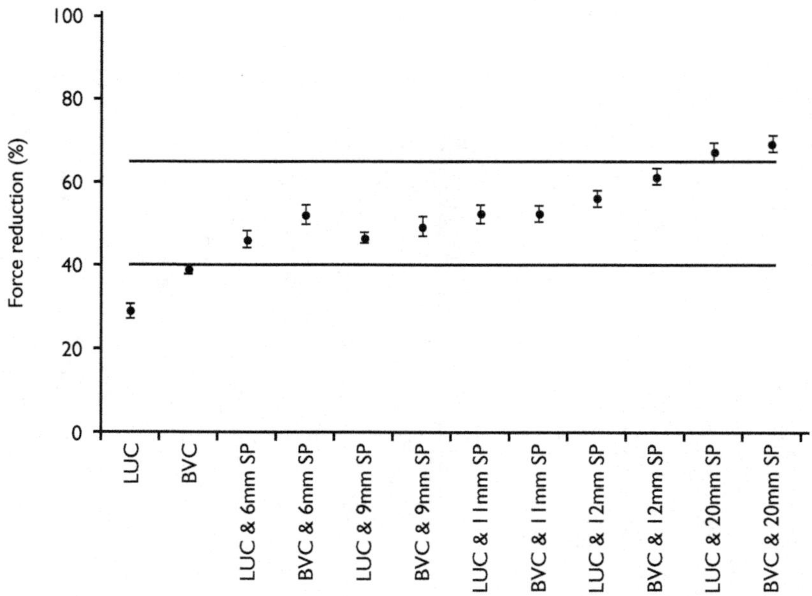


*Figure 3.10* A graph to show the mean force reduction (%) measured by the Artificial Athlete on 12 artificial hockey carpet/shockpad systems of varying type and thickness (on a concrete floor in a laboratory). LUC = 11mm nylon carpet with a 3mm integral shockpad and BVC = 11mm nylon carpet with 6mm integral shockpad, with increasing thickness of a separate shockpad (SP) beneath. The data whiskers show 1 standard deviation, and the horizontal lines show the 40 and 65 per cent limits for FIH 'national'-level approval. See Table 3.2 for detail. (Reproduced from Young, 2006, with permission.)

*al*., 2011; Saunders *et al*., 2011; Fleming, 2011b) as a faster and simpler measure of hardness than the AA or AAA, or through lack of availability of the standard AA or AAA. The Clegg measures the peak deceleration using an accelerometer attached to the impacting mass. The readout device displays the peak value, in units of gravities (9.81ms$^{-2}$). It has been demonstrated to produce useful correlations with the AA/AAA regarding force reduction on point elastic sports surfaces such as long-pile rubber-filled carpets (Fleming, 2011b; Young, 2006; Severn, 2010) but poor correlation on sand-filled (e.g. hockey) surfaces (Young, 2006). The Clegg hammer has been proposed as a useful tool for site monitoring of hardness via its simple method, whereby if the surface system becomes progressively harder the Clegg reading may increase to a trigger value whereby a more detailed investigation is then required or a specific maintenance (e.g. a decompaction) process. It is noted that in Australia the 2.25kg Clegg hammer appears in the AFL guidelines for ground hardness safety for natural turf and artificial turf standards, as explained on its community football website (AFL, 2012, 2013).

A separate test is used to assess the potential for a user's head injury, commonly called the 'HIC' or 'head injury criterion'. The test data can also be interpreted as the 'critical fall height' (EN 1177, 2008). This test method appears in several IGB standards in relation to rugby (union and league), for indoor sports hall floors and in Australian Rules football (AFL, 2012) and was first introduced as part of the UK's standards for playground surfaces hence the term 'critical fall height'. The principle is that as the drop height of a rigid falling mass increases so too does the peak deceleration. A maximum level of peak deceleration (i.e. 200 ms$^{-2}$) permitted can be expressed as the critical fall height of a surface. The standard defines the impact attenuation property of a surface as the property which dissipates the kinetic energy of an impact by localised deformation or displacement such that the (peak) acceleration is reduced. The 'critical fall height' is defined as the 'maximum free height of fall, for which a surface will provide an acceptable level of impact attenuation'. It defines the head injury criterion (HIC) value as a criterion for head injuries caused from falls, linked to severity of potential damage to the brain.

The apparatus comprises a rigid hemispherical head form of 160mm diameter and a mass of 4.6kg incorporating an accelerometer. A useful review of the potential for head injury on long-pile rubber infill surfaces for soccer is given in Theobald *et al.* (2010), showing a comparison between artificial turfs in comparison to high-quality natural turf. The shockpad and sand-rubber infill were identified as key components in maximising the impact attenuation properties. The impact attenuation of all the tested artificial turfs was found to be independent of moisture content, and hence safety levels remained consistent in both arid and extremely wet conditions, according to the study.

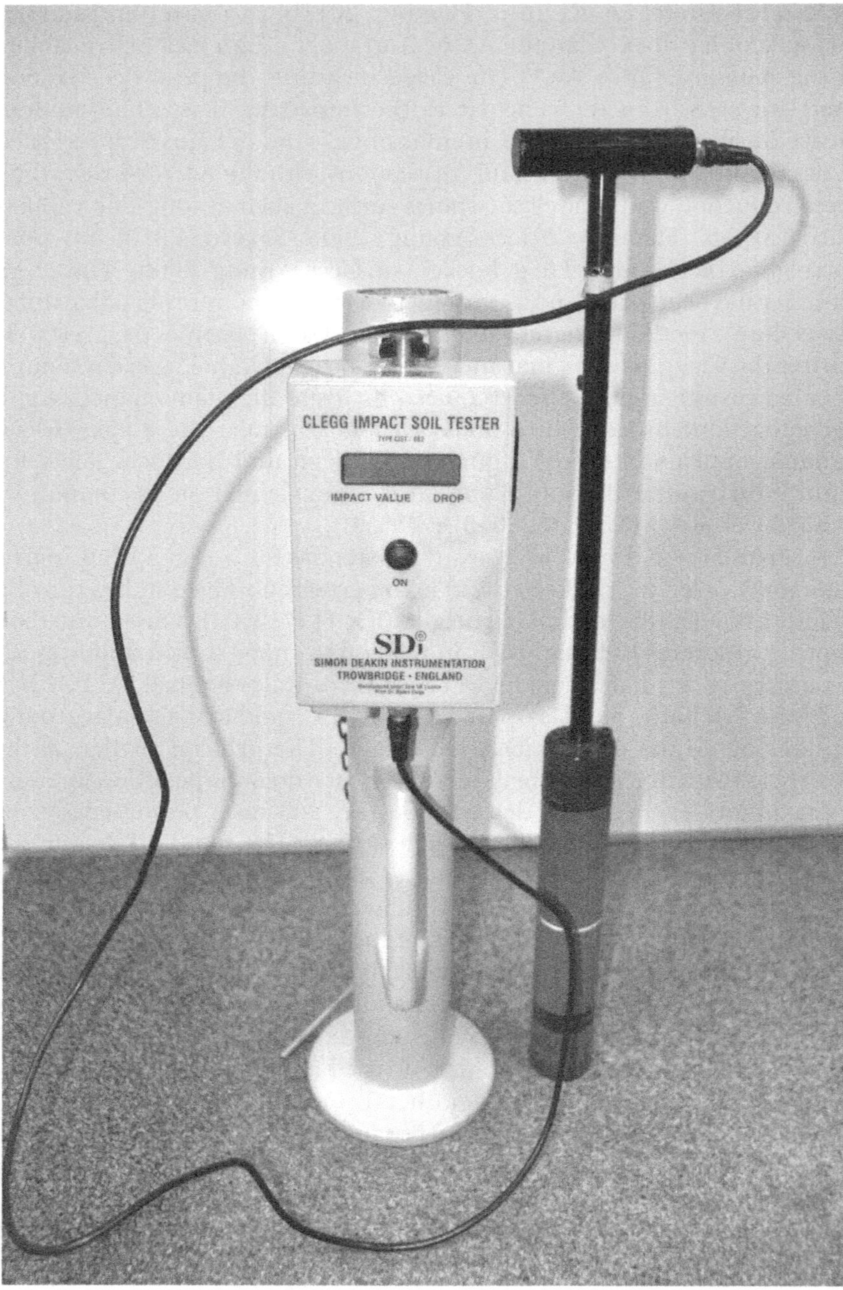


*Figure 3.11* Picture of the Clegg Impact Hammer (2.25kg version) showing the drop hammer separate to the guide tube. The readout box is held in the operator's hand during the drop test (personal photograph).

The rugby codes' guidance stipulates that a shockpad is required to pass this 'head' impact test. The guidance further permits a slight reduction in the minimum drop height value (to achieve a peak deceleration of 200g $ms^{-2}$) in the field after two years to reflect an expected hardening of the surface system with time (World Rugby, 2012), e.g. from ≥1.3m to ≥1.0m.

### *Tests relating to friction/traction*

Sports players use specific footwear with studs (termed cleats in some countries) or spikes to penetrate and interlock with the playing (or running) surface, and generate resistance which is usually termed 'traction' force. This ability to generate traction between a player's footwear and a sporting surface is a crucial factor influencing the player's movement and performance. The traction force produced contributes to the locomotion of an athlete and their ability to change velocity (accelerate or decelerate), and to change direction, or in the case of rugby help generate scrummage forces between the teams. The level of traction produced at the shoe–surface interface reportedly has the potential to contribute to or cause injury, whereby too low a traction resistance force will result in slipping, while excessive traction resistance may cause foot 'sticking' to occur (FIFA, 2012a). In addition, resistance to a player sliding bodily on a surface, whereby discomfort and abrasion burns can result, became a topic of great interest to both the players and the governing bodies, particularly for soccer and the sliding tackle manoeuvre, with the advent of longer and softer-pile carpets in the 1990s, discussed further below.

#### *Shoe–surface traction tests*

The standards for shoe–surface grip were borne originally from the test method for slip resistance in use for many years for factory floors and roofs to ensure workers' safety. The slip resistance test uses a simple pendulum device fitted with a specified rubber contact strip fixed to the swinging test 'foot'. In principle it measures the energy loss of the swinging pendulum after the test foot contacts with the floor/surface (BS EN 14837, 2006). This standard was itself derived from the highway industry whereby the portable pendulum test was developed to estimate the 'skid resistance' of a road surface (BS EN 14231, 2003) by measuring the surface friction (see Figure 3.12). This test is used widely within the sports surface industry, and has been adapted in several ways to improve its usefulness on the longer-pile turfs by adding studs, for example, and also by measuring the initial deceleration of the foot as it makes contact with the surface. The mass of the swinging arm and studded test foot is specified as 2kg. The pendulum test measures translational friction, i.e. in one plane, and measures only dynamic friction, albeit it is not a constant velocity test. The test foot can be varied for different sports such as soccer and hockey.

Specific to sports surfaces, a rotational traction test device was also developed based on work in the 1980s at the Sports Turf Research Institute wherein test methods and performance limits were identified for natural and artificial turf (Baker, 1989). The device comprises a simple studded disc, rotated by the operator using a calibrated torque wrench and the maximum resistance torque is recorded. The FIFA test method specifies the rate of rotation as 12 revolutions per minute (manually controlled by the operator) and a minimum angle of rotation as 90 degrees (i.e. the test should take approximately 1–2 seconds). The test foot uses a standard equal spacing of six football studs for soccer and rugby, adapted to other stud patterns to suit hockey or a dimpled sole used for cricket (see Figure 3.13). A static mass of 46kg is stipulated for the test, which renders it less portable, and in some cases the test procedure requires the mass to be lifted and dropped from 60mm to assist in stud penetration. In general, too high a value of rotational traction is said to represent the possibility of 'foot lock' and potential ankle injuries (Shorten *et al.*, 2003).

There exists a clear difference between the simple translational and rotational traction-related tests described above and the more complex player movement (Fleming, 2011b). These tests measure in principle the maximum dynamic traction resistance for specific boundary conditions of the tests and at the laboratory-prepared, or field state, of the surface, which is in essence unknown. The traction resistance required by a player/athlete for movement performance and to protect safety is however a complex issue with many interacting variables and the reader is directed

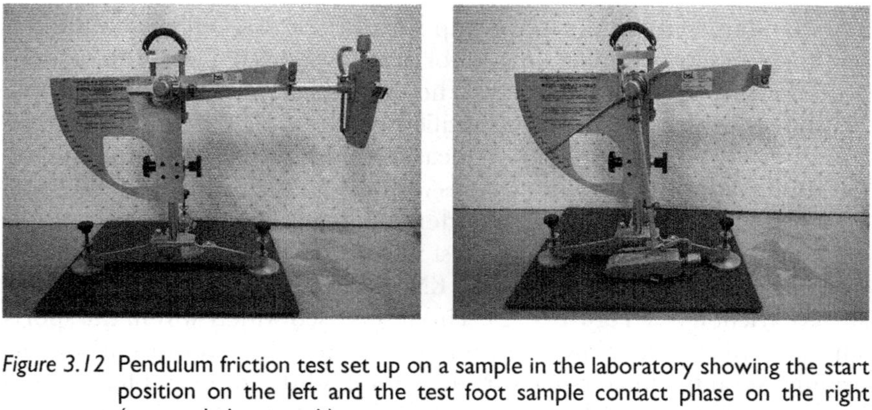

*Figure 3.12* Pendulum friction test set up on a sample in the laboratory showing the start position on the left and the test foot sample contact phase on the right (personal photograph).

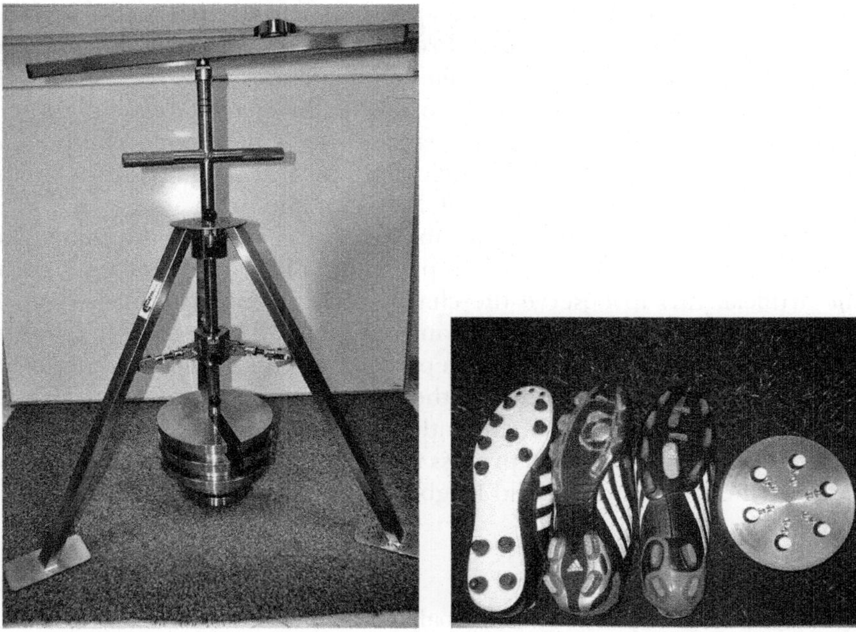

*Figure 3.13* Rotational traction tester showing the apparatus set up on a sample on the left and the underside of the six-studded base plate on the right, next to some boot outsoles for comparison (personal photograph).

to Chapters 4, 5 and 7 for further information regarding the biomechanics of human movement on surfaces, injury risks and research into performance, and Chapter 6 for a fuller review of the science and research into mechanical shoe–surface interaction.

### *Skin friction test*

The advent of artificial turf raised an interesting issue in player feedback regarding skin burns and abrasions, which were reportedly higher on artificial turf than natural turf (Fuller *et al.*, 2007). While early generations of artificial turf utilised abrasive fibres (nylon in particular), the longer-pile (third-generation) turfs introduced in the 1990s are comprised of polypropylene and polyethylene and designed to provide lower skin abrasion.

In response to player feedback, a test method was developed specifically for football (FIFA, 2012a) termed the 'securisport' skin friction tester. This test comprises an apparatus that controls the rotation of a simple test foot onto which a silicon 'skin' is mounted and the resistance to rotation is measured to determine the coefficient of friction at the interface. The method requires calibration of the apparatus and specialist silicon 'skin' samples which have to be changed regularly. The test method stipulates that a vertical force of 100N is applied to the test foot in contact with the turf sample and five revolutions are made at a speed of 40 revolutions per minute. The mean horizontal resistance force is determined and from this the mean coefficient of (dynamic) friction. It is repeated three times with new silicon 'skin' and new infill in the sample.

The test is also used to estimate abrasion, by comparing the change in coefficient of the virgin silicon sample from before and after testing on the artificial turf to observe the change using a smooth polished steel plate (with a known very low friction coefficient). The change in friction of the silicon 'skin' is expressed as a percentage and a limit of 30 per cent change is permitted – related to the wear caused by the artificial turf sample. The test method is currently applied only in the laboratory as part of the product approval process within World Rugby, RFL and FIFA performance standards (World Rugby, 2012; RFL, 2011; FIFA, 2012b).

### *Ball–surface interaction*

The fundamental behaviour of a ball–surface interaction involves some complexity to analyse it analytically. For this reason the general approach taken in standards relating to ball behaviour is to utilise simple empirical tests that, in general, link to in-play performance. Football and hockey have relatively simple ball bounce and ball roll tests that indirectly measure, or are influenced by, surface hardness and surface friction (see Tables 3.1 and 3.2).

However, the ball and surface can deform upon contact, such that energy losses are affected by both the ball and surface stiffness and damping properties. It has been shown that the rebound behaviour (often termed the coefficient of restitution, the ratio of rebound velocity to impact velocity) is influenced by drop height such that the standards specify a drop height and an envelope of acceptable rebound heights for the surface to be deemed acceptable (EN 12235, 2013). The ball pressure, if pressurised, is crucial and its direct measurement is problematic, so usually a rebound height test is performed on 'concrete' or a similar rigid surface to meet a stipulated rebound height and the ball pressure adjusted as required.

Ball roll on outdoor pitches is affected by external effects such as wind and surface wetness. For these reasons field testing often specifies a maximum wind speed, and that roll tests are done in four directions at 90 degrees to each other and averaged. The averaging of the directional tests can also eliminate bias and systematic error from the surface having directional properties such as orientation of fibres, or from a slope on the surface (required for drainage reasons for example). Furthermore, spin can exert an influence on the interaction with regard rebound height and angle of rebound, and this adds complexity for repeatability of tests. For this reason apparatus that fire balls such as cannons or simple drop tests are required to deliver no spin to the ball before contact with the surface (e.g. angled ball behaviour test BS EN 13865 [2003]).

It is also apparent that the balls used for the simple drop and roll tests should conform to a specific standard themselves. The governing bodies' websites should be consulted for further details on this topic, however in principle ball-related standards include specifics on ball size, sphericity, weight and may also include stipulation of the component materials and deformation properties.

Tennis has a relatively long history, in comparison to other sports, of strict guidelines and approval processes for ball approval for tournaments and these requirements appears to have been fixed since 1996 (ITF, 2012). The international tennis governing body (ITF) introduced a relatively sophisticated 'surface pace' test method to rate a court surface, with five categories from 'slow' through to 'fast'. This was, it seems, in relation to concerns over the game of tennis increasing in (ball) pace during play through improvements in racquet performance (lighter, stiffer composites) and player performance (strength and technique). In the ITF surface pace test (see ITF CS 01/02, ITF 2012) a tennis ball is fired at high velocity of around $30 ms^{-1}$ (without spin) at a low angle (16 degrees) of incidence, to replicate a typical 'hard' service, and the rebound velocity and height are measured and combined to give both an estimate of surface friction and a 'surface pace' rating. The inclined surface pace test requires a ball cannon and light gates to measure velocity and velocity changes. The FIFA quality concept includes an angled ball rebound test in their requirements for lab testing with a soccer ball but is not a requirement for field testing (this was originally in place but was removed in 2012). This also applies for rugby union (using a soccer ball). Hockey has discussed and debated the merits of a similar test for its specification apparently but have yet to introduce it formally.

## *Discussion of performance-related testing*

The test methods described in the previous sections represent the industry-recognised test standards and governing-body specifications that enable comparison between surface systems and provide a set of tools to implement the guidelines on pass/fail criteria for components and/or the surface system (for product approval and installation). In general the test methods and specifications have been predicated to provide 'safe' surfaces and provide adequate performance and skill associated with the sport in question. Whether the tests can be improved and whether they provide realistic simulations of player movement or ball interactions can be debated, on several levels. It is also important to consider that once a surface system is installed it will deteriorate through mechanical wear and environmental ageing processes. Thus its performance and safety risks will change.

However, assessment or evaluation of the safety and injury risks of surface systems for the users is complex, and has not been studied in detail directly in epidemiological research. User performance in relation to optimising movement efficiency or for the use of equipment on the surface (such as the ball) has also not been studied in great detail to date. Chapters 4, 5 and 7 deal with the issues of player movement and performance in more detail.

The test methods in current use by the sport governing bodies were developed empirically and have evolved in recent years into well-regulated procedures. The general philosophy of the governing bodies in comparing say artificial turf to natural grass, or comparing performance between established surface types to new ones, is in general a sound principle. This approach is somewhat constrained, however, in that it does not address the important questions regarding how the surface properties may actually influence performance or injury risk, and therefore does not strive to provide a route to improve the safety of surfaces (Shorten, 2010). It also appears appropriate to suggest that most of the current test methods are rather simple in order to provide repeatable measurements that are easy to interpret. If the aim of a test method was to simulate human movement, by providing more dynamic loading for example, the test devices would necessarily become more complex, more costly and commercially less attractive to developers and manufacturers. Thus it is perhaps incumbent on the research community to develop more advanced knowledge of sports surfaces to explain response behaviour and to develop more sophisticated test methods to measure the multivariate interaction of player–surface mechanisms of traction or impact loading, for example. Frequently, however, coupled to increased complexity of mechanical testing comes non-standardisation of both the methods of measurement and data analysis and interpretation with regard the potential effects for the user. There currently exists no agreed standard method for preparing surface samples for testing in research or for reporting of the sample 'state' (or any changes in state that may occur during testing). Addressing these issues is an ongoing challenge.

As an example of the surface behaviour challenges in both deriving test methods and reporting them, the behaviour under compressive loading can be considered. When one considers the effect of the (vertical) impact force applied to the materials under test and their likely response, particularly those strain hardening (see Figure 3.14) elastomeric materials such as rubber particulate and foams (used widely in sports surfacing products), the material stiffness response is clearly dependent on the initial state and also the load path length (i.e. applied load magnitude). As a consequence, there is a need to carefully set the mechanical test load magnitude (and contact area) to produce the most appropriate material response in relation to the expected response under an athlete's loading. Furthermore, the hysteresis behaviour of the materials under test, i.e. energy loss through deformation, is a function of the strain levels induced and hence a product of the magnitude of stress applied and the material stiffness response to that stress level. The application of inappropriate loads (and contact area) in mechanical testing will lead to 'incorrect' material responses for deformation and strain, energy loss and energy return in relation to what may be expected for the human loading scenario. The multilayer (and thin layer) construction of most modern sports surface systems leads to further exacerbation of these challenges of interpreting impact test data, for example, as the impact response will depend on the stress and strain distribution in possibly all of the layers. The effect of load direction further exacerbates this mismatch between some mechanical testing and human loading.

It is the authors' opinion that to enhance the further development of mechanical tests more 'in-game' loading measurements from players/ athletes during their interaction with surfaces is required. This data could, with some consensus, be used to develop a useful 'state-of-the-art' database. This would enable the enhanced development or modification

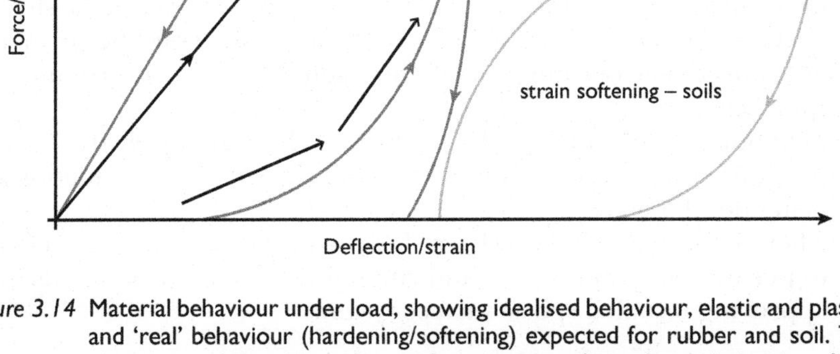


*Figure 3.14* Material behaviour under load, showing idealised behaviour, elastic and plastic, and 'real' behaviour (hardening/softening) expected for rubber and soil. The two stress path vectors (arrows) attempt to show the variation in rubber stiffness response (non-linear strain hardening) expected for the same stress tensor but different initial conditions whereby when already under some compression/load there is a higher stiffness response.

of current test devices to more closely recreate these recognised loading conditions and contribute to more reliable testing procedures. There is also scope to utilise the players themselves as the test devices if consensus on movement types, measurement and analysis systems were harmonised. In addition, and concurrently, a separate strand of research is required that moves the science forward in both measuring and modelling surface behaviour under load and its 'ageing' process. Studies that measure the response of the system, at a suitable level of detail for each of the respective component's behaviour, is required for the development and validation of numerical modelling of sports surface systems. The development of suitable predictive models will enable studies into rapidly determining the likely effects of material and/or system design changes, and coupled to biomechanical models permit the 'virtual' prediction of the interaction loading effects on the user for estimating performance and/or safety.

## Key summary points

- Sports surfaces should meet a list of requirements. Key ones include: be of consistent quality and performance at installation and during serviceable lifetime; provide safe interaction for users in normal use; provide appropriate ball interaction performance; and not adversely affect the local environment.
- Testing of surfaces should be routinely used for approval and to demonstrate the requirements set out in quality assurance systems.
- A wide array of standards and specifications exist, covering mechanical testing methods and targets for compliance in relation to categories of player–surface interaction, ball–surface interaction and durability. These standards do not (yet) comprise any testing using players as subjects.
- International sports governing bodies specify quality assurance procedures for product acceptability and also for installed surface systems, stipulating acceptable performance limits. These performance limits in some cases differentiate between elite level and community sport level.
- Maintenance of surfaces is required. Through applied research programmes test methods to better quantify surface degradation are being developed.
- There exists a gap in knowledge between user movement in relation to performance and injury, and current mechanical testing aimed at approving installed sports surface systems.

## References


Australian Football League (AFL) (2012) *Preferred Facility Guidelines for State, Regional and Local Facilities*. Online. Available at: www.aflcommunityclub.com.au/index.php?id=891 (accessed 09/04/2013).

Australian Football League (AFL) (2013) *Artificial Grass for Sport Guide*. Online. Available at: www.aflcommunityclub.com.au/index.php?id=891 (accessed 09/04/2013).

Baker, S. W. (1989) 'The playing surface characteristics of natural turf and synthetic turf surfaces for association football', *Journal of Sports Science*, 62: 9–35.

BS 7044-1 (1990) *Artificial Sports Surfaces – Part 1: Classification and General Introduction*. London: BSI.

BS EN 1177 (2008) *Impact Attenuating Playground Surfacing. Determination of Critical Fall Height*. London: BSI.

BS EN 12235 (2013) *Surfaces for Sports Areas. Determination of Vertical Ball Behaviour*. London: BSI.

BS EN 13865 (2003) *Surfaces for Sports Areas. Determination of Angled Ball Behaviour*. London: BSI.

BS EN 14231 (2003) *Natural Stone Test Methods. Determination of the Slip Resistance by Means of the Pendulum Tester*. London: BSI.

BS EN 14808 (2005) *Surfaces for Sports Areas – Determination of Shock Absorption*. London: BSI.

BS EN 14809 (2005) *Surfaces for Sports Areas – Determination of Vertical Deformation*. London: BSI.

BS EN 14837 (2006) *Surfaces for Sports Areas. Determination of Slip Resistance. Status*. London: BSI.

BS EN 14877 (2013) *Synthetic Surfaces for Outdoor Sports Areas – Specification*. London: BSI.

BS EN 14904 (2006) *Surfaces for Sports Areas – Indoor Surfaces for Multi-use Sports – Specification*. London: BSI.

BS EN 15301-1 (2007) *Surfaces for Sports Areas. Determination of Rotational Resistance*. London: BSI.

BS EN 15330-1 (2013) *Surfaces for Sports Areas – Synthetic Turf and Needle Punched Surfaces Primarily Designed for Outdoor Use – Part 1: Specification for Synthetic Turf*. London: BSI.

BS EN 15330-2 (2008) *Surfaces for Sports Areas – Synthetic Turf and Needle Punched Surfaces Primarily Designed for Outdoor Use – Part 2: Specification for Needle-Punched Surfaces*. London: BSI.

English Cricket Board (ECB) (2007) *TS6 – Technical Requirements and Performance Specification for Non-Turf Cricket Pitches*. Online. Available at: www.ecb.co.uk/development/facilities-funding/facilities-guidance-and-project-development (accessed 09/04/2013).

FIFA (2012a) *Quality Concept for Football Turf, Handbook of Requirements*. Online. Available at: www.fifa.com/mm/document/footballdevelopment/footballturf/01/13/56/09/fqchandbookoftestmethods(january2012).pdf (accessed 10/09/2012).

FIFA (2012b) *Quality Concept for Football Turf, Handbook of Test Methods*. Online. Available at: www.fifa.com/mm/document/footballdevelopment/footballturf/01/13/56/08/fqchandbookofrequirements(january2012).pdf (accessed 10/09/2012).

FIH (2014) *The Handbook of Performance Requirements for Synthetic Turf Hockey Pitches Incorporating Test Procedures*. Online. Available at: www.fih.ch/en/fih/sport/pitches (accessed 09/06/2014).

Fleming, P. R. (2011a) 'Maintenance best practice and recent research', *Proceedings of the Institution of Mechanical Engineers, Part P, Journal of Sports Engineering and Technology*, 225(3): 159–170.

Fleming, P. R. (2011b) 'Artificial turf systems for sport surfaces: Current knowledge and research needs', *Proceedings of the Institution of Mechanical Engineers, Part P, Journal of Sports Engineering and Technology*, 225: 43–64.

Fuller, C. W., Dick, R. W., Corlette, J. and Schmalz, R. (2007) 'Comparison of the incidence, nature and cause of injuries sustained on grass and new generation artificial turf by male and female football players. Part 1: match injuries', *British Journal of Sports Medicine*, 41: 120–126.

IAAF (2008) *IAAF Track and Field Facilities Manual*. Online. Available at: www.iaaf.org/about-iaaf/documents/technical#certification-system.

ITF (2012) *Approved Tennis Balls, Classified Surfaces and Recognised Courts 2012 – A Guide to Products and Test Methods*. Online. Available at: www.itftennis.com/technical/home.aspx (accessed 12/12/2012).

James, I. T. and McLeod, A. J. (2010) 'The effect of maintenance on the performance of sand-filled synthetic turf surfaces', *Sports Technology*, 3(1): 43–51.

Jan-Kieft, G. (2009) *Quality Monitoring of 50 Artificial Turf Fields. Presented at the SportSURF Seminar on 'Maintaining performance of synthetic surfaces'*. Online. Available at: http://sportsurf.lboro.ac.uk (accessed 23/02/2012).

Joosten, T. (2003) *Players' Experiences of Artificial Turf*. Presented at Stadia Turf Summit, Amsterdam. Online. Available at: www.isss-sportsurfacescience.org/downloads/documents/6EGR67DKG1_Joosten.pdf (accessed 10/09/2013).

McLaren, N. J., Fleming, P. F. and Forrester, S. E. (2012) 'Artificial grass: A conceptual model for degradation in performance', 9th International Sports Engineering Conference, Boston, MA, *Procedia Engineering*, 34: 831–836.

McLeod, A. (2008) *The Management and Maintenance of Second Generation Sand-Filled Synthetic Sports Pitches*, Engineering doctorate thesis, Cranfield University, UK, 2008. Online. Available at: http://dspace.lib.cranfield.ac.uk/handle/1826/2625.

Rugby Football League (RFL) (2011) *Performance and Construction Standards for Synthetic Turf Rugby League Competition and Training Pitches*. Online. Available at: www.rflfacilitiestrust.co.uk/_uploads/RFL%20Performance%20Standard%20for%20synthetic%20turf%20pitches%20(11-10-11).pdf (accessed 12/08/2013).

Saunders, N., Twomey, D. and Otago, L. (2011) 'Clegg hammer measures and human external landing forces: Is there a relationship?', *International Journal of Sports Science and Engineering*, 5(4): 231–236.

Severn, K. S. (2010) *Player Surface Interactions: Traction on Artificial Turf*, PhD thesis, Department of Civil and Building Engineering, Loughborough University.

Shorten, M. R. (2010) 'Sports surfaces and injury: the missing link', Proceedings of the Second International Conference on Science, Technology and Research in Sport Surfaces, Loughborough, UK, April, Loughborough University

Shorten, M., Hudson, B. and Himmelsbach, J. (2003) 'Shoe–surface traction of conventional and in-filled synthetic turf football surfaces', Proceedings of the

15th International Congress of Biomechanics, University of Otago, Dunedin, New Zealand (eds P. Milburn *et al.*), p.6.

Sport and Play Construction Association (SAPCA) (2009) *The SAPCA Code of Practice for the Construction and Maintenance of Synthetic Turf Sports Pitches,* 3rd edition, SAPCA, January 2009. Online. Available at: www.sapca.org.uk/default (accessed 20/12/2012).

Sport England (2007) *Floors for Indoor Sports: Design Guidance Note*. London: Sport England.

Sports Council (1984) *Specification for Artificial Sports Surfaces*. London: Sport England.

Theobald, P., Whitelegg, L., Nokes. L., Chatur, Z. and Jones, M. (2010) 'The predicted risk of head injury from fall related impacts on to 3rd generation artificial turf and grass soccer surfaces: A comparative biomechanical analysis', *International Journal of Sport Biomechanics*, 9(1): 29–37.

Tipp, G. and Watson, V. J. (1982) *Polymeric Surfaces for Sport and Recreation*. London: Applied Science.

Twomey, D., Otago, L., Ullah, S. and Finch, C. F. (2011) 'Reliability of equipment for measuring ground hardness and traction', *Journal of Sports Engineering and Technology*, 3: 131–137.

Young, C. (2006) *Performance of Water-based Hockey Pitches*, PhD thesis, Department of Civil and Building Engineering, Loughborough University.

World Rugby (2012) *Regulation 22 – Standard Relating to the Use of Artificial Rugby Turf*. Online. Available at: www.irbplayerwelfare.com/ (accessed 01/03/2013).

World Rugby (2013) *Natural Surfaces – Section G 'Equipment'*. Online. Available at: www.irbplayerwelfare.com/ (accessed 12/02/2013).

Chapter 4

# Sports surfaces, biomechanics and injury

*Victoria Stiles and Sharon Dixon*

## Introduction

Playing surface characteristics are often associated with injury, with surface friction and hardness being the two main features most frequently implicated (Ekstrand and Nigg, 1989; Milburn and Barry, 1998; Nigg and Segesser, 1988; Rogers and Waddington, 1990; Bastholt, 2000; Orchard *et al.*, 2008). It is likely that the loading of structures within the body will change for surfaces with different cushioning or friction characteristics. In addition, the properties of a playing surface may change the fundamental technique utilised by a player to perform a task. For example, they may perform faster on a harder surface, or change their movement pattern when turning on a surface that allows sliding compared to one with high resistance to sliding. These differences are likely to influence the loading on structures of the body and thus the likelihood of injury. However, there is little direct evidence to support this suggestion.

While surface characteristics are often suggested to be associated with injury risk, little is understood regarding the mechanisms by which injury risk varies dependent on the characteristics of a surface. This chapter considers biomechanical mechanisms for injury risk on surfaces with different characteristics. The chapter evaluates evidence regarding: 1) the influence of surface characteristics on injury incidence; 2) the influence of surface characteristics on biomechanical measures; and 3) the association between biomechanical measures and injury. Evidence from each of these areas is brought together to inform our understanding of mechanisms of injury with changing surface characteristics (Figure 4.1). Future directions for investigating associations between sports surfaces and injury mechanisms including player perceptions are also explored.

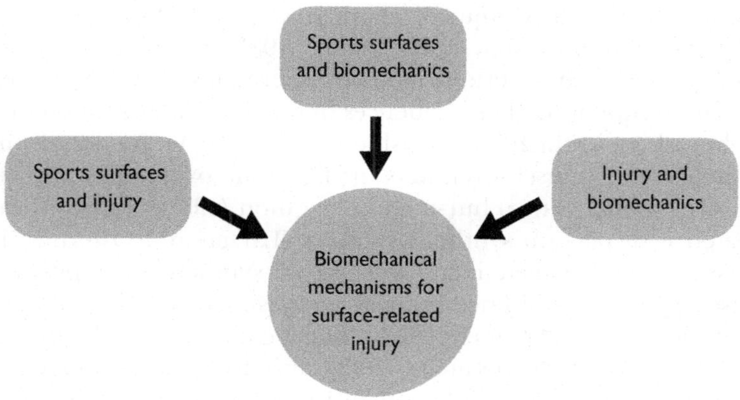


*Figure 4.1* Illustration of suggested approach to developing relationships between sports surfaces, biomechanics and injury to infer injury mechanisms.

## Do the playing surface characteristics influence injury incidence?

This section evaluates evidence associating sports surface characteristics with injury incidence and type. There is a focus on field sports, tennis and running, owing to the predominance of relevant studies being in these sports.

### *Field sports*

#### *Early generations of synthetic turf*

As outlined in previous chapters, synthetic turf pitches were developed to provide an all-weather alternative to natural turf, which also allowed repeated training and matches without the recovery time required for natural turf pitches. These surfaces have been designed to replicate the properties of natural turf pitches and can be used around the clock, resulting in an increase in pitch use. While the initial introduction of synthetic sports surfaces led to an increase in the number and frequency of people involved in sport, there was also a documented increase in the type and frequency of injury (Nigg and Yeadon, 1987; Dragoo and Braun, 2010).

Early generations (first and second) of synthetic sports surfaces, characterised by high levels of stiffness, sliding traction and heat retention (Keene *et al.*, 1980) with flaking turf fibres creating debris that packed the surface and increased its hardness (Bowers and Martin, 1974), were associated with skin abrasions, lower leg pain ('shin splints'), Achilles tendinopathy and knee injuries (Torg *et al.*, 1974; James *et al.*, 1978; Andreasson and Olofsson, 1983; Nigg, 1983; Clement *et al.*, 1984; McCarthy, 1989). In American football, where falls on flexed knees and elbows are frequent, higher incidences of bursitis (inflammation of fluid-filled bursal sacs which help cushion and alleviate friction from the movement of skin, muscles, tendons and ligaments over bone), particularly of the pre-patellar (knee) bursa and olecranon (elbow) bursa, were also associated with play on synthetic surfaces (Larsen and Osternig, 1974). The association between increased use of synthetic turf pitches and increased prevalence of knee injuries such as medial collateral ligament and anterior cruciate ligament (ACL) damage in American football in the 1980s (Powell and Schootman, 1992) also likely contributed to the reluctance of soccer codes of football to embrace early generations of synthetic turf. Additionally, synthetic turf at this time resulted in balls bouncing higher and rolling faster (Keene *et al.*, 1980), thus changing the playing characteristics of the game compared to natural turf surfaces. Differences in surface hardness and frictional properties of early-generation synthetic surfaces compared to natural turf were speculated to contribute to the differences in injury (Orchard *et al.*, 2005).

### *Natural versus third-generation turf*

As outlined in Chapter 2, the 1990s saw the development of third-generation synthetic turf, with longer pile length than previous generations and the use of sand/rubber granule infill. Comparisons of injury incidence between natural turf and third-generation turf in football codes of sport are popular owing to the use of both surface types in training and matches.

To assess how common an injury is, injury occurrence is typically presented as an incidence ratio, providing a relative measure based on the number of injuries per thousand hours of exposure (Hodgson-Phillips, 2000). Injury incidence during training and match play has been found to be similar between third-generation synthetic turf and natural turf surfaces (Fuller *et al.*, 2007a; 2007b; Steffen *et al.*, 2007; Ekstrand *et al.*, 2011; Soligard *et al.*, 2012). However, differences in the type of injury most commonly experienced by soccer players during matches and training on natural and synthetic turf surfaces have been reported (see Table 4.1). In summary, Fuller and colleagues found that for men, knee ligament tears, particularly of the ACL, were the most common season-ending injury during training and matches on natural turf, whereas tears to the hamstring and lateral ankle ligament were the most common season-ending injuries on synthetic turf during matches and training respectively (Fuller *et al.*, 2007a, 2007b). For women, knee ligament tears, particularly of the ACL, have been reported to be the most common season-ending injury on natural and synthetic turf during both matches and training (Fuller *et al.*, 2007a, 2007b).

While the most common season-ending injuries tend to be to the knee, ankle ligament tears are the most commonly reported injury for both men and women. For men, they occur more frequently during matches (Ekstrand *et al.*, 2011) as well as being the most common season-ending injury during training on synthetic turf (Fuller *et al.*, 2007b). Conversely, a higher incidence of ankle ligament injury was found for women on natural turf compared to synthetic turf during matches (Fuller *et al.*, 2007a). A meta-analysis of injury incidence for third-generation synthetic turf surfaces relative to natural turf found that six out of fourteen cohorts revealed a beneficial effect on the occurrence of muscle injuries when playing on synthetic turf (Williams *et al.*, 2011). However eight cohorts revealed an increased risk of incurring an ankle injury when playing on synthetic turf (Williams *et al.*, 2011).

The body of available research comparing injury incidence on third-generation and natural turf surfaces suggests that while the overall incidence of non-contact lower limb injuries between these surfaces is similar, injury type whether season-ending or otherwise, may differ between surfaces and between sexes, and may also be influenced by match-play and training (Fuller *et al.*, 2007a, 2007b; Bjørneboe *et al.*, 2010; Ekstrand *et al.*, 2011). However, a consistent evidence-based conclusion regarding an elevated or reduced risk of injury when playing on synthetic or natural turf remains to be found. Caution is also advised when interpreting injury pattern data due to some studies having low sample sizes and exposure times, particularly for female datasets. This leads to low levels of statistical power from which only cautious conclusions can be drawn. In addition, both natural and third-generation turf surfaces have quite variable properties, with these properties typically poorly quantified in injury studies.

### *Tennis*

High levels of pain, specifically foot pain and lower limb injury, are reported by tennis players (Nigg *et al.*, 1986). Compared to other sports, the repetitive side-to-side movements in tennis have been associated with high incidences of specific conditions including plantar fasciitis and tendinopathy of the Achilles, posterior tibial and flexor hallucis tendons (Lynch and Renström, 2002). The twisting and turning movements in tennis also subject the knee to a variety of varus/valgus alignments, flexion-extension movements and internal or external rotations. These movements result in repeated and sometimes excessive strains and stresses leading to knee pain, meniscus tears, patellar tendinitis and knee ligament injuries (Renström and Lynch, 2002).

*Table 4.1* Most common lower limb injuries during match play and training for men and women playing soccer on natural turf and third-generation artificial turf.

| | Natural turf | | Artificial turf | | Reference |
|---|---|---|---|---|---|
| | Men | Women | Men | Women | |
| **Most common season-ending injuries** | | | | | |
| Matches | ACL tears | ACL tears | Hamstring tears | ACL tears | Fuller *et al.*, 2007a |
| Training | Knee ligament tears | Knee ligament tears | Ankle ligament tears* | Knee ligament tears | Fuller *et al.*, 2007b |
| **Most common injuries (1 = highest incidence)** | | | | | |
| Matches | 1. Ankle lateral ligament complex tear<br>2. Hamstring tear | 1. Ankle lateral ligament complex tear*<br>2. ACL tear | 1. Ankle lateral ligament complex tear<br>2. Hamstring tear | 1. Ankle lateral ligament complex tear<br>2. ACL tear | Fuller *et al.*, 2007a |
| | 1. Hamstring strain<br>2. Ankle sprain | 1. Ankle sprain<br>2. Hamstring strain | 1. Ankle sprain*<br>2. Hamstring strain | 1. Ankle sprain<br>2. Hamstring strain | Ekstrand *et al.*, 2011 |
| Training | 1. Ankle lateral ligament complex tear<br>2. Hamstring tear | 1. Ankle lateral ligament complex tear<br>2. Quadriceps tear | 1. Ankle lateral ligament complex tear<br>2. Quadriceps tear | 1. Ankle lateral ligament complex tear<br>2. Hamstring tear | Fuller *et al.*, 2007b |
| | 1. Hamstring strain<br>2. Ankle sprain | 1. Hamstring/ quadriceps/ calf strain | 1. Ankle sprain<br>2. Hamstring strain | 1. Ankle sprain<br>2. Hamstring strain | Ekstrand *et al.*, 2011 |

* Indicates within a gender and injury type a significantly higher incidence of injury compared to the other surface ($p<0.01$).

As detailed in Chapter 2, tennis is played on a variety of surfaces around the globe, including hard courts, grass and clay. The two main surface types that offer the most insight in terms of injury incidence and biomechanical response are acrylic hard courts and traditional red clay courts, owing to their distinctly different hardness and friction properties. Acrylic hard courts were originally introduced in the 1940s and comprised an asphalt or concrete base overlaid with a rubber shock-absorbing layer coated with acrylic/polyurethane paint. These surfaces provide the stiffest surface in tennis yielding a high ball-bounce and the highest player–surface frictional coefficient as a result of the rough paint finish. The high coefficient of friction enables players to experience a greater rate of acceleration and deceleration compared to play on clay (Girard *et al.*, 2007). This explosive style of play has been suggested to explain the higher incidence of plantar fasciitis, joint hyperextension and muscle fatigue seen on this surface (Lynch and Renström, 2002). More incomplete matches (which are normally terminated due to player injury) were observed on US hard courts for men and Australian hard courts for women compared to all other surfaces (Cross, 2006). This is consistent with anecdotal reports of an association between increased levels of pain in recreational and professional tennis players as a result of playing on hard courts compared to more forgiving, low-friction surfaces such as clay (Nigg and Segesser, 1988).

'Clay', which has been popular since the 1950s, especially in European countries, consists of crushed stone layers topped with fine gritty clay (Miller, 2006). It is generally assumed to cause fewer injuries compared to hard courts due to low levels of sliding friction (Bastholt, 2000; Miller, 2006). Significantly fewer medical treatments were reported for professional players when playing on clay compared to grass and hard courts (Bastholt, 2000). Lower levels of knee injury were also observed for senior players who played predominantly on clay throughout their tennis lives (Kulund *et al.*, 1979). However, compared to hard courts, the slower-paced clay courts with lower coefficients of friction are associated with higher incidence of muscle strains and spasms. This has been suggested to be a result of the tibialis posterior and calf muscles, in particular, working to stabilise joints during sliding (Lynch and Renström, 2002). The introduction of 'blue clay' at the Madrid Open in 2012 caused new controversy with reports of a lack of control over sliding and stopping (BBC Sport, 2012). This suggests that if the use of alternative clay surfaces such as 'blue clay' continues, the performance and injury parameters for these models of clay court may be different to that of traditional red clay.

In addition to mechanical properties of a surface, monitoring of playing style may offer insight into the different patterns of injury for each surface. On clay, playing style typically involves more lateral movements along the baseline, longer exchanges, greater foot sliding and higher ball bounces. This is compared to a more aggressive style on grass, with little or no foot sliding and lower ball bounces that often pick up speed after surface contact (Bastholt, 2000). Hard courts have been observed to yield a combination of clay and grass-court playing styles as a result of hard, rough surfaces resulting in longer rallies without the option to slide easily (Bastholt, 2000).

Comparisons between synthetic and natural turf data for soccer (Ekstrand and Nigg, 1989) and American football (Torg *et al.*, 1974), suggest that players who frequently change from one surface to another may be at a higher risk of incurring injury (Williams *et al.*, 2011). This may have implications for injury incidence in tennis where elite players perform competitively with relatively little time to adjust to frequent changes in surface. In light of these suggestions and with support from players, changes have been made to the Grand Slam calendar, with the Wimbledon Championships 2015 commencing one week later than previously to allow players more time to adjust from the clay court final of the French Open at Roland Garros and utilise a longer grass-court preparation phase in the run-up to Wimbledon.

### Running

Running surfaces can include any surfaces available in the local environment, and thus typically include asphalt, concrete, grass, trails (grass/soil/gravel), sand, running tracks and treadmills. Anecdotally, there are frequent suggestions of the running surface type being influential on injury. However, there is little, if any, scientific evidence to support this association. For example, a study of over 800 runners training for a 10km race over 13 weeks reported no association between running terrain (road, trail, grass, track and treadmill) and the number of injuries experienced (Taunton *et al.*, 2003). Interpretation of the findings of such studies is complicated by the difficulties in accurately quantifying the time spent running on each surface type and the intensity of training for each surface. Rather than controlling the specific running surfaces used, athlete reporting is relied upon. Ideally a randomised controlled trial would be utilised to administer surface types in a controlled manner, but the challenges involved in such a study design mean that this study has not yet been performed.

For competitive track and field events, surface hardness is the aspect of track design that has been most frequently implicated regarding injury risk. Running track design has developed with a focus on performance, primarily for the sprint events. As described in Chapter 2, early competitive running tracks were constructed from cinder, and were relatively soft and forgiving, but required regular levelling and were influenced dramatically by weather conditions. 'All-weather' polyurethane 'Tartan' track surfaces were developed in the 1960s by the company 3M, with the 1968 Summer Olympics in Mexico seeing the first synthetic track being used for Olympic competition. Modern running tracks typically comprise a polyurethane or latex layer, providing a relatively uniform surface and being usable in all but the most extreme weather conditions. The focus on performance has led to the development of relatively hard surfaces at the elite level, with injury implications rarely considered. This was highlighted by the example of the 1996 Atlanta Olympic Games, where several distance runners complained that the track was too hard. Most notably, following heats and final in the 10,000m event, Haile Gebrselassie withdrew from the 5,000m event, reportedly due to the unacceptable hardness of the track. As highlighted in Chapter 3, the international governing body of athletics (the IAAF) has regulations regarding the track shock-absorption, utilising mechanical test procedures to provide a range for force reduction permitted for track surfaces (range: 35–50 per cent). The track at Atlanta was measured as having 36 per cent force reduction, placing it at the upper limit of hardness acceptable for international competition at the time (Dixon *et al.*, 2000), thus supporting the suggestions of athletes that the track felt hard.

While there are clear mechanical differences in both the cushioning and traction provided by different running tracks, scientific evidence regarding relationships with injury is lacking. Messier *et al.* (1995) reported a greater amount of track running to be associated with the development of iliotibial band syndrome, although the authors acknowledge that it was not possible to distinguish between the effect of the running track itself (mechanical properties) and the type of training performed. For example, interval type training, with fast bouts of running, is typical when training on a running track, compared with more steady-state running on other surfaces. The act of running bends on the track may also influence injury risk, with asymmetries in muscle strength being reported for track runners (Beukeboom *et al.*, 2000).

The studies outlined so far usefully describe associations between the incidences of injury and changes in surface for different sports. However they rarely examine the cause and effect relationship between identified risk factors and specific types of injury. Increased knowledge of surface-related mechanisms of injury is required to develop models of player–shoe–surface interaction to improve surface and player performance and reduce the risks of acute and overuse injury. One approach to investigate mechanisms of injury is to relate observed differences in injury risk to changes in biomechanics for different surfaces.

## Are biomechanical measures influenced by changes in surface characteristics?

The differences in injury incidence suggested by the results of injury studies are likely to be the result of variations in mechanical characteristics of the surfaces, primarily differences in surface friction and/or hardness (Ekstrand and Nigg, 1989; Milburn and Barry, 1998; Nigg and Segesser, 1988; Rogers and Waddington, 1990; Bastholt, 2000; Orchard *et al.*, 2008). Although it is difficult to isolate the effect of changing friction or hardness when comparing sports surfaces, with both likely changing to some extent, typically a comparison of surfaces will involve a change where adjustment of either friction or hardness is dominant. For example, when comparing running on concrete or on natural turf, there will be differences in both mechanical friction at the shoe–surface interface and in surface hardness, but the difference in hardness is likely to be dominant. In this section, while acknowledging that both generally change to some extent, evidence for surface cushioning and traction influencing biomechanical measures is presented. Evidence is derived from studies of running and of movements typical for soccer and tennis. More detailed evaluation of changes in biomechanical measures for different sports surfaces is provided in Chapter 7.

### *Cushioning*

The resultant ground reaction force (GRF) between the human and the ground during sports movements can be quantified using a force platform (see Chapter 7). The peak rate at which vertical force is applied (peak rate of loading), represented by maximum steepness of the vertical force curve during the ascending impact phase (see Figure 4.2) in the first 50ms of ground contact has been suggested to be a reliable indicator of loading underfoot with changes in shoe (Clarke *et al.*, 1983a, 1983b; Hennig *et al.*, 1996) and surface (Stiles and Dixon, 2007) mechanical cushioning.

Peak rates of loading for young adult females (18–25 years) during running on a concrete floor at a relaxed pace are typically in the range 30–40 bodyweights (BW) per second (Lilley *et al.*, 2011). During a sport-specific movement such as the foot plant of a tennis running forehand on a concrete floor (Figure 4.2), peak rate of loading for a similar age group has been measured as approximately 360 BW/s (Stiles and Dixon, 2006). Dixon and Stiles (2003) reported no change in peak loading rate when running on tennis surfaces with different levels of cushioning. In contrast, comparison of loading rate during a running forehand foot-plant revealed significant differences (Stiles and Dixon, 2006). Thus, differences in GRF loading rate may be detected for changes in playing surface, but it is important to use sport-specific movements yielding realistic loading magnitudes to determine the extent of these effects.

Pressure data provide detail regarding the distribution of vertical load across the foot/shoe plantar surface (see Chapter 7). For tennis, analysis of loading under foot using pressure insoles during tennis-specific movements has revealed that hard courts yield significantly higher loading of the hallux (big toe) and lesser toes compared to clay (Girard *et al.*, 2007). In contrast, relative loads under the medial and lateral mid-foot were higher on clay compared to hard court, suggested by the authors to be a result of different playing styles (Girard *et al.*, 2007). It was suggested that players are more aggressive utilising front-foot landing strategies on hard courts compared to more defensive responses and a deep baseline playing position on clay. On clay, this allows increased time for players to respond using more sliding, side-to-side steps that exert pressure through the mid-foot (Girard *et al.*, 2007).

Analysis of pressure insole data has also revealed differences in loading beneath the foot on third-generation synthetic compared with natural turf for sport-specific movements. Total loading under the foot has been found to be similar with changes in turf, suggested to indicate that synthetic turf can replicate overall loads typically found on natural turf (Ford *et al.*, 2006). However, when analysing the distribution of pressure under regions of the foot, peak pressures under the medial aspect of the foot were found to be significantly higher on natural turf compared to

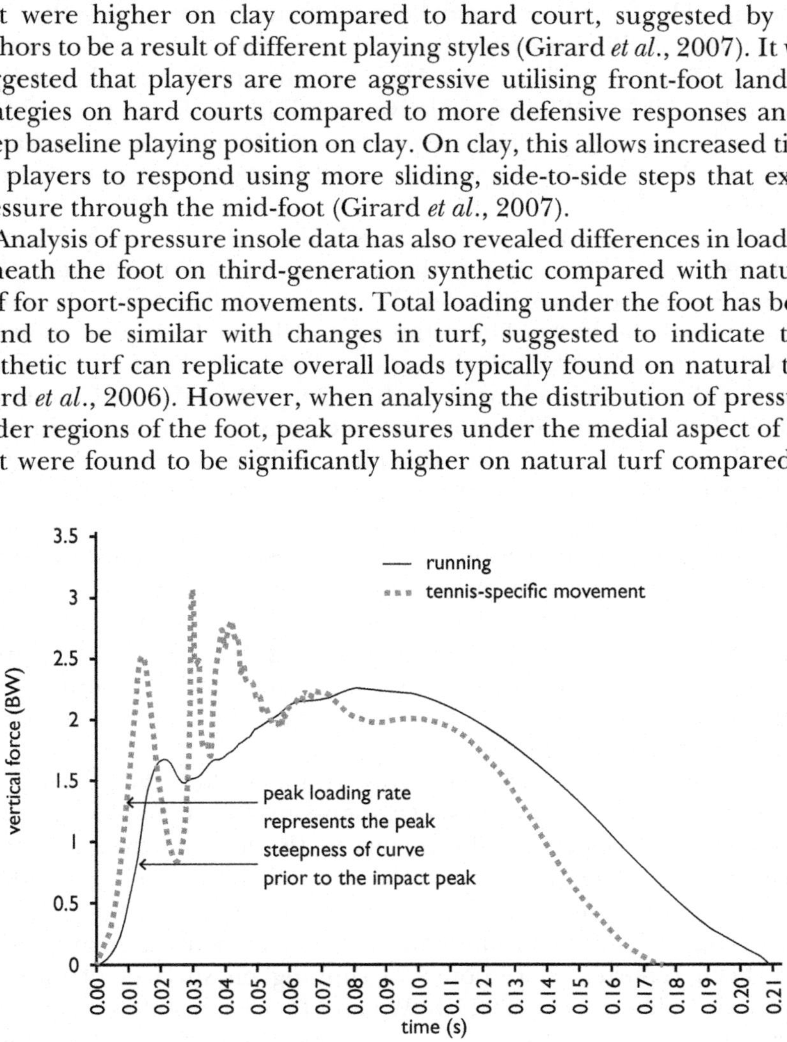


*Figure 4.2* Typical vertical force-time histories for running and tennis running-forehand foot-plant, identifying the peak loading rate (steepness of the curve) for each movement.

third-generation synthetic turf. The authors suggested that increased medial pressures during cutting may be caused by increased rigidity of natural turf supporting the medial foot (Ford *et al.*, 2006).

In-shoe pressure data have also been compared for different surfaces during running. For example, Wang *et al.* (2012) demonstrated significant differences in plantar pressures for concrete, synthetic rubber and grass. In particular, the grass surface resulted in lower pressures at several areas of the foot and also increased ground contact time when compared with concrete. This evidence would help us to understand possible injury mechanisms if differences in injury incidence were recorded for running on these different surface types. However, this injury information is not currently available. While speculative, an additional factor to consider is that harder surfaces may improve performance by allowing faster running times, but that this greater speed may itself increase injury risk (Norton *et al.*, 2001).

While force plate and pressure insole data provide some indication of biomechanical changes with variation in sports surface, these measures do not provide detail on the loading experienced by structures of the body. The estimation of lower limb joint moments provides an indication of changes in function about the different joints, although limitations must be acknowledged (see Chapter 7). Data collected in our laboratory have demonstrated increases in initial dorsi-flexor moment and in peak plantar-flexor moment during the midstance phase of running for concrete compared with foam (Figure 4.3). These observations suggest a greater use of the tibialis anterior to control rapid plantar-flexion of the foot following initial heel strike, and also a greater use of the calf muscles (gastrocnemius and soleus) during propulsion, for the harder surface condition. Estimating lower limb joint moments in response to changes in surface conditions therefore provides further scope for increasing understanding of how athletes respond to changes in surface that might influence surface-related mechanisms of injury.

There is also some evidence that runners alter their lower limb movement patterns (kinematics) in response to changes in playing surface characteristics. Kinematic adjustments in the form of increased initial knee flexion (cushioning flexion), reduced heel impact velocity, reduced initial foot sole angle relative to the horizontal (increasing the area of the foot in contact with the ground) and variations in joint angular velocities have been reported in response to running on surfaces of increased hardness (Bobbert *et al.*, 1992; De Wit and De Clercq, 1997; De Wit *et al.*, 2000; Dixon *et al.*, 1998; Dixon *et al.*, 2000). In terms of sport-specific movements, a reduced fifth metatarsal-phalangeal (MTP) joint impact velocity has been found during turning on a natural turf surface, which was the hardest study condition with the highest resistance to shear failure

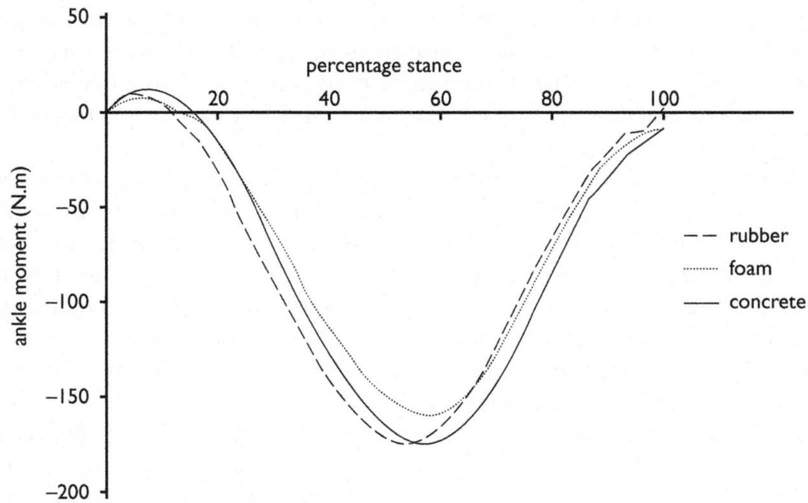


*Figure 4.3* Sagittal plane ankle moment time histories when running on surfaces of differing stiffness.

(Stiles *et al.*, 2011). It is noted that the ability to detect kinematic response to changes in playing surface when studying sport-specific movements is complicated by the variety of techniques used to accomplish a movement task. In addition, the closed, non-negotiable performance of a skill has been suggested to prioritise consistent production of a movement (outcome-orientated movement) regardless of variations in surface properties. This may explain the absence of kinematic response to significant changes in impact interface in some studies of sport-specific movements (Stiles and Dixon, 2007). Experience of negative sensory input as a result of harder surfaces may trigger impact-moderating kinematic responses during open movements such as running. However changes in lower body kinematics during sport-specific, task-orientated movements may be detrimental to the outcome, explaining the minimal kinematic responses observed (Hamill *et al.*, 1999; Shorten, 2000).

### Friction

The peak horizontal force measured by a force plate can be used to indicate the shear requirements of a surface for different movements. In field sports played on natural turf, which 'gives' and moulds in response to loading, participants wearing studded footwear were found to yield peak horizontal forces in the region of 0.6 bodyweights when accelerating from rest (Stiles *et al.*, 2009) and 0.9 bodyweights during turning (Stiles *et al.*, 2011). This compares with running on a natural turf surface yielding approximately 0.2 bodyweights of horizontal force during the braking phase (Stiles *et al.*, 2011). The comparison of typical horizontal force-time histories in Figure 4.4 (in direction of travel) indicates that accelerating and turning movements make greater use of the shear properties of turf compared to running.

As well as presenting the vertical and horizontal components of ground reaction force separately, force plate data have been used to provide a utilised coefficient of friction, determined by the ratio of peak horizontal force to peak vertical force (see Chapter 7). As an example of how the coefficient of friction changes with courts in tennis, Stucke and colleagues found that accelerating from rest on a hard court yielded a coefficient of friction of 0.90, indicating a high level of static friction, compared to 0.65 on cinder, a sliding surface (Stucke *et al.*, 1984).

Differences in lower limb joint moments have also been detected for changes in playing surface frictional properties. A greater internal knee adduction moment (muscle moment tending to adduct the knee) was observed for a tiled surface permitting horizontal movement compared with non-sliding surfaces (Nigg *et al.*, 2009). In contrast, for a shoe–surface combination with low resistance to sliding, a lower internal knee adduction moment was reported than for a shoe–surface interaction with high resistance to sliding (Dowling *et al.*, 2010). This difference between studies

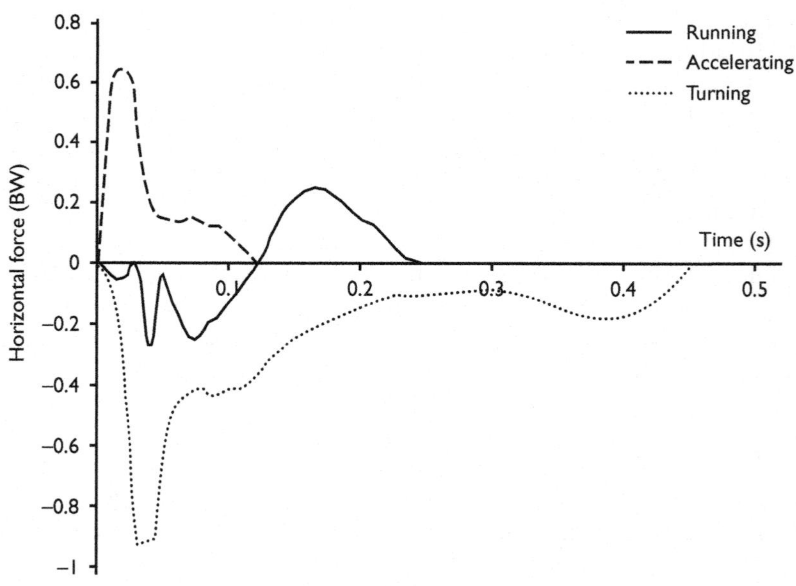


*Figure 4.4* Comparison of typical anterior-posterior horizontal force–time histories for accelerating from rest, turning and running on natural turf wearing studded footwear.

is most likely a result of the different mechanisms employed to allow horizontal movement of the shoe, with the sliding of the shoe over the surface in the work described by Dowling *et al.* (2010), compared with movement of the tiled surface and shoe combination in the study of Nigg and colleagues (2009).

Comparison of court surfaces at opposite friction extremes has demonstrated differences in kinematics during a stopping movement in tennis. In this example, the knee joint continued to flex when stopping on the hard court (high friction) as an unloading mechanism compared to a fixed angle of knee flexion when sliding on a cinder court (Stucke *et al.*, 1984). Kinematics during initial ground contact have also been reported to be influenced, with a high-friction surface yielding lower magnitudes of initial knee flexion during turning compared with a low-friction surface (Dowling *et al.*, 2010). This evidence of differences in kinematics highlights the variation in technique necessary when playing tennis on surfaces with differing levels of friction.

Evidence from studies of natural turf also supports this suggestion that players adjust movement patterns in response to changes in surface properties. An integrated biomechanical and engineering study of natural turf surfaces found that varying the mechanical hardness and shear strength of natural turf by changing the contribution from clay, sand and silt components within ryegrass-turfed root-zones influenced lower limb kinematics during soccer-specific movements (Stiles *et al.*, 2011). During turning movements, the horizontal (direction of run-up) and resultant impact velocities of the fifth metatarsal-phalangeal joint (fifth MTP) were found to be significantly lower for a 'clay' condition (hardest surface with the greatest resistance to shear failure) compared to a sand/clay turf condition (least hard surface with moderate shear strength). A reduction in the impact velocities of the foot when contacting the hardest surface with the greatest shear strength indicates that this measure is sensitive to changes in mechanical properties of the impact interface, contributing to our increased understanding of player–shoe–surface interaction during sport-specific movements.

This summary of biomechanical changes for varying surface characteristics, particularly cushioning and traction, highlights the potential of surfaces to influence movement and loading. But are these biomechanical changes influential on injury?

## Do changes in biomechanics influence injury risk?

This section considers evidence regarding whether the changes observed in human biomechanics with changing playing surface characteristics are influential on injury risk.

Measurements of ground reaction force have revealed associations with injury in some studies. For example, in a retrospective study of runners, those with a history of lower limb overuse injury were found to have greater loading rate of GRF than uninjured runners (Hreljac *et al.*, 2000). In prospective studies, high loading rates of GRF have been associated with tibial stress fracture in female runners (Grimston *et al.*, 1991; Milner *et al.*, 2006). There is also evidence of greater loading rate of GRF in those with knee pain (Radin *et al.*, 1991). While there are also studies that have failed to link this variable with lower limb injury (Crossley *et al.*,1999; Bennell *et al.*, 2004), the balance of evidence suggests that loading rate of GRF may be an important variable to measure when comparing different sports surfaces biomechanically.

Measurement of pressure distribution across the foot plantar surface has also revealed associations with injury. Both Willems *et al.* (2005) and Rice *et al.* (2013) have performed prospective studies where individuals with relatively high pressure at the medial forefoot during propulsion have been reported to be at increased risk of experiencing an ankle inversion injury. A prospective study of military recruits in training has reported greater forefoot pressures for individuals prone to metatarsal stress fracture (Nunns, 2014).

As previously indicated, measurement of joint moments provides an estimate of changes in internal load. In runners, the frontal plane knee moment applied over time (angular impulse) has been associated with the development of patellofemoral pain (Stefanyshyn *et al.*, 2006). Greater internal knee abductor moments have been associated with increased localised loading and cartilage deterioration in the knee joint (Bennell *et al.*, 2010), and with the development of medial knee osteoarthritis (Miyazaki *et al.*, 2002). These findings suggest that changes which influence joint moments, such as differences in surface, are likely to influence joint loading and thus the risk of injury and possible development of osteoarthritis.

Biomechanical variables associated with the specific injury of ACL rupture have been investigated quite extensively owing to the high prevalence of this injury in sports (Griffin *et al.*, 2006; Orchard *et al.*, 2008; Yu and Garrett, 2007). The occurrence of non-contact ACL injuries has been associated with excessive tension in the ligament as a result of activities involving sudden deceleration, landing and pivoting movements (Griffin *et al.*, 2006; Yu and Garrett, 2007;) particularly when the foot remains fixed to the floor (Olsen *et al.*, 2003). A small knee flexion angle (especially during landing), a strong muscular contraction from the quadriceps and a greater posterior (braking) ground reaction force (GRF) that increases the tendency for anterior translation of the tibia, are considered important mechanisms for elevating ACL loading and injury risk (Griffin *et al.*, 2006; Yu and Garrett, 2007). During a stop-jump task, increases in the posterior GRF have been found to directly result in a greater force of contraction from the quadriceps (disproportionate to the force of hamstring contraction) which increases ACL loading (Yu *et al.*, 2006). Therefore, individuals experiencing greater posterior GRFs during athletic tasks are believed to be at a higher ACL injury risk (Yu and Garrett, 2007).

Overall, this evidence regarding biomechanical risk factors for injury has highlighted that surface characteristics that influence loading, as detected by measures of ground reaction force, plantar pressures, joint angles and/or joint moments, may influence the risk of injury when performing on a particular surface. We therefore have evidence that some aspects of surface design can influence injury incidence, that key biomechanical measures can be changed by a manipulation in surface, and that some of these biomechanical measures have been associated with injury. The challenge is to bring evidence from each of these areas together to develop suggested mechanisms by which changes in surface influence injury risk (Figure 4.1).

## Suggested biomechanical mechanisms for surface-related injury

In this section, evidence from the three areas of: a) sports surfaces and injury; b) sports surfaces and biomechanics; and c) injury and biomechanics, are brought together to suggest biomechanical mechanisms for surface-related knee and ankle injuries (Figure 4.1).

### *Knee injuries*

Knee pain associated with overuse conditions such as patellofemoral pain syndrome and patellar tendinitis has been associated with increased shoe–surface friction (Renström and Lynch, 2002). In addition, changes in shoe–surface friction have been found to be influential on knee ab/adductor moment, although the direction of change depends on the properties of the shoe–surface combination (Nigg *et al.*, 2009; Dowling *et al.*, 2010). It is therefore suggested that the mechanism by which changes in friction of the shoe–surface interface influence knee injury is through an effect on the internal knee adductor moment (indicative of a change in knee joint loading), but that the specific effect (increase or decrease in loading) should be investigated for the shoe–surface combination of interest.

Differences in shoe–surface friction are also the most frequently suggested reason for differences in the incidence of acute knee ligament injury across surfaces. High shoe–surface traction or increased form-locking (penetration of surface by footwear) have been reported to result in high horizontal (braking) ground reaction forces (Stiles *et al.*, 2009).

High braking forces have also been associated with increased knee ligament tension (Yu *et al.*, 2006), thus providing a suggested mechanism for increased knee ligament injury risk for high friction conditions. This foot fixation mechanism for ACL injury through high braking force most likely combines with knee flexion and knee internal rotation to misalign the knee medially (knee valgus), as indicated by the increased internal knee adductor moment observed for high friction conditions (Dowling *et al.*, 2010). These links between ACL injury and surface–player interaction have been made most frequently for synthetic football (soccer) turf surfaces, but are also relevant to other sports surfaces where movements with high braking forces occur such as in landing and turning.

Although high shoe–surface friction is often associated with synthetic compared with natural turf surfaces, characteristics of natural turf may also lead to high friction. On a natural turf pitch, friction is additionally influenced by soil type, soil density, grass root density and soil moisture content, meaning that variations in the type of natural turf are likely to influence injury risk (Stiles *et al.*, 2009). Thus, associations between high shoe–surface friction and increased injury risk have also been suggested to explain differences in knee ligament injury across different types of natural turf. For example, Bermuda grass has been suggested to increase the incidence of knee ligament injuries as a result of it yielding higher shoe–surface traction compared to perennial ryegrass as a result of the growth structure of this grass containing horizontally creeping stolons which form a mesh near the top of the surface, increasing resistance to wear but also increasing traction (Canaway *et al.*, 1990; Orchard, 2001; Orchard *et al.*, 2005) (see Chapter 8 for more detail).

Constructing a natural turf pitch from portable square systems has been additionally implicated regarding ACL injury risk (Orchard *et al.*, 2008). Such a construction necessitates the use of grasses such as Kentucky bluegrass, to provide lateral growth to hold the grass cover together. However it also results in high levels of mechanical traction that produce an increased form-locking effect with studded footwear, thus increasing braking forces. Similarly, the synthetic reinforcement of soil material to reduce surface wear using polyester nylon meshes near the soil surface has also been linked with increased risk of knee joint injuries as footwear become locked in the mesh (Orchard, 2002).

Thus, both synthetic and natural turf surfaces have characteristics that may influence the level of friction and thus the risk of injury. For both surface types, awareness of the specific shoe–surface combination is important for determining the effect on knee joint loading. For natural turf, the grass type, coupled with poor installation and pitch inconsistency, may also play a significant contribution to knee ligament injury in field sports, particularly when played on portable grass systems (Orchard *et al.*, 2008).

### Ankle inversion injury

We have highlighted ankle inversion injury as common in sports participation, with some evidence that surface characteristics are influential. High medial forefoot pressures during running have been associated with increased susceptibility to this injury (Willems *et al.*, 2005; Rice *et al.*, 2013). Changes in forefoot pressure have also been observed for different surface conditions. Specifically, Ford *et al.* (2006) observed greater medial forefoot pressures when performing cutting steps on natural compared with synthetic turf. This is consistent with the observed greater incidence of ankle inversion injury on natural compared with synthetic turf for females during match play (Fuller *et al.*, 2007a). This may suggest a mechanism for this different injury incidence through greater medial forefoot loading during sports movements, although does not explain the contrasting reports of greater incidence of ankle inversion injury on synthetic turf for males. An alternative mechanism is suggested by the results of a study of the volley in tennis, where hard court surfaces were associated with a tendency for greater lateral pressures, suggesting the rear foot is in a more inverted orientation (Girard *et al.*, 2007). This may increase the risk of ankle inversion injury on harder surfaces for these types of sport-specific movement.

### Exercise-induced lower leg pain (EILLP)

While evidence is limited, an increased incidence of lower leg pain, including medial tibial stress syndrome and tibial stress fractures, has been associated with harder playing surfaces, in particular during the transition period from a clay court to a harder surface in tennis (Lynch and Renström, 2002). Peak loading rate of ground reaction force and peak heel pressures have been reported to be greater for surfaces with greater stiffness/hardness (Stiles and Dixon, 2006; Wang *et al.*, 2012). In addition, peak loading rate has been linked with risk of tibial stress fracture, and aspects of plantar pressure have been associated with EILLP (Milner *et al.*, 2006; Willems *et al.*, 2007). Greater dorsi-flexor and plantar-flexor moments have also been reported for harder surface conditions, suggesting an increased loading of lower leg structures (see Figure 4.3). Together, these observations provide some evidence that increases in overuse injuries of the lower leg associated with harder running/playing surfaces are a result of greater loading of the lower limb.

The combined evidence regarding biomechanical measures associated with injury risk and with changes in surface has allowed the suggestion of mechanisms for development of some types of injury on surfaces with specific characteristics. However, such suggestions remain speculative and are based on limited evidence. To strengthen these links, studies are required in which injury, biomechanics and surface characteristics are measured simultaneously.

## Player perceptions of changes in surface

In the previous section, speculative associations relating surface characteristics, biomechanics and injury have been made through the approach outlined in Figure 4.1. This approach is useful in terms of highlighting important aspects of surfaces and biomechanics. One aspect that has not been considered so far is that of player perception of the surface characteristics and the influence this may have on the biomechanical response of the player and thus the risk of injury. To successfully interact with any environment, sensory input is continuously processed by an individual and interpreted in relation to previous experience and memories to inform individualised perceptions (Coren *et al.*, 1979; Fleming *et al.*, 2005; Visell *et al.*, 2011). Perceptions influence and control human movement, helping us interact with surfaces in our environment (Visell *et al.*, 2011). Perception of surface cushioning and frictional properties make important contributions to player–shoe–surface interaction, however a variety of more subtle interactions are available during sports performance that have a bearing on these responses.

Following Fleming and colleagues' work on player perceptions of synthetic surfaces in hockey (Fleming *et al.*, 2005), tennis player perceptions captured using visual analogue scales and semi-structured interviews with changes in surface have been compiled using thematic analysis (Starbuck *et al.*, 2011). A range of responses were identified demonstrating how players understand, interpret and attach meaning to changes in mechanical properties of a court surface. The main perceptions based on surface 'predictability', 'hardness' and 'grip' were informed by sub-themes including 'player–surface interactions', 'ball–surface interactions', 'performance', 'injury' and 'playing environment' (Starbuck, unpublished PhD research). Player perceptions to changes in mechanical properties of a tennis court are being studied alongside biomechanical responses (e.g. pressure underfoot, lower limb kinematics) and adjustments in technique employed on different surfaces to further develop models of player–shoe–surface interaction.

In soccer, feedback from players indicates they tend to prefer to play on natural turf rather than synthetic turf, indicating that attitudes may need to be reconsidered in order for players to fully embrace modern synthetic turf pitches (Dick *et al.*, 2003). Anecdotal opinions from soccer players performing on natural and synthetic turf (undisclosed type) indicated that players preferred natural turf, perceiving that impact was reduced (supported by mechanical test data), ball roll was slower and the surface was more comfortable to play on (supported by reduced heat retention and improved moisture retention) compared to synthetic turf (Martinez *et al.*, 2004). Leg and muscle problems were also perceived by players to be less on natural turf compared to synthetic turf (Martinez *et al.*, 2004).

While the negative perceptions of increased incidence of injury when playing on early generations of synthetic turf may be reconsidered in relation to third-generation pitches, differences in playing characteristics such as fewer sliding tackles and more shorter passes on third-generation synthetic turf continue to influence player attitudes and reinforce their overall negative impression towards synthetic turf (Andersson *et al.*, 2008). Elite male soccer players also reported that ball control was poorer when playing on third-generation synthetic turf compared to natural turf and perceived that a greater physical effort was required on synthetic turf despite time-motion analysis revealing similar activity intensities for each surface (Andersson *et al.*, 2008). In contrast, five-a-side recreational soccer players commented that playing on a surface with higher stiffness and friction (asphalt) was less demanding (lower level of perceived exertion) compared to playing on a surface with lower surface stiffness and friction (synthetic turf) despite similar total distances covered during each game (Brito *et al.*, 2012). These perceptions were supported by significantly lower mean heart rates and a smaller percentage of total playing time spent above 90 per cent of the maximum heart rate on asphalt compared to synthetic turf, even though asphalt yielded an increased number of high-intensity runs (sprints) compared to synthetic turf (Brito *et al.*, 2012).

## Final remarks

A range of both natural and synthetic surfaces are being used for sports participation. Surface design is increasingly sport-specific which, together with the development of player-, sport- and surface-specific shoes, has resulted in models of player–shoe–surface interaction becoming highly specialised (see Chapter 7). To optimise performance while reducing injury risk, the surface layer in particular must be considered from both engineering and player perspectives. Figure 4.5 depicts the feedback loops necessary to develop an acceptable surface, taking into account the effect of changes in properties of the surface and the player including performance and injury perspectives. Models of player–shoe–surface interaction and surface development therefore rely on knowledge of surface-related injury incidence, developments in surface engineering (performance and sustainability) and biomechanical risk factors for

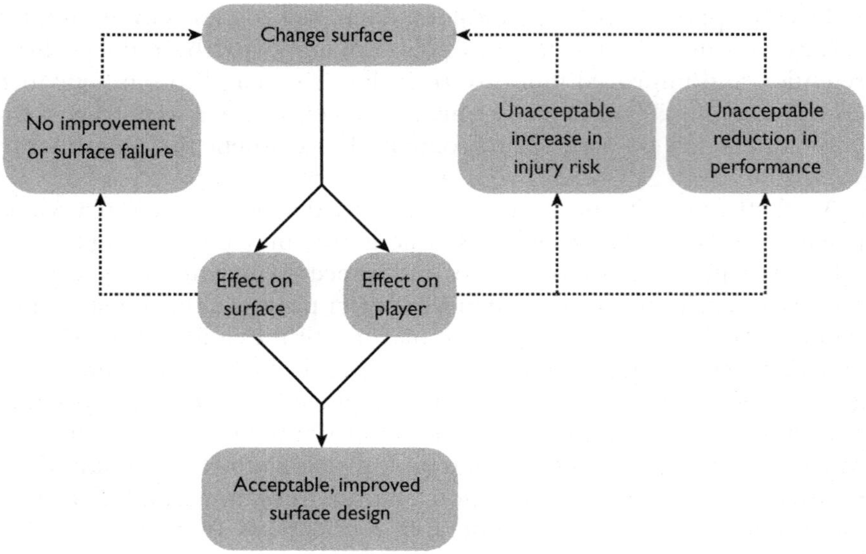


*Figure 4.5* Integrated engineering and biomechanical approach to sports surface development to optimise surface performance standards while reducing surface-related injury risk. Reproduced from Stiles *et al.*, 2009, with permission from Adis (© Springer International Publishing AG 2009. All rights reserved).

injury. These models could also be extended to include player perceptions and attitudes towards surface performance.

To fully develop and appreciate the depth and breadth of how humans respond to changes in impact interface, contributions from all areas of sports science and surface engineering are required. An integrated approach involving measures from biomechanics, psychological perspectives (perception), sports medicine and surface engineering will increase knowledge of player–shoe–surface interaction and inform the future development of sports surfaces that optimise performance and minimise injury risk.

In sports with varying surface type, research is needed to: a) characterise how player technique adapts to changes in the shoe–surface combination (Fleming *et al.*, 2005; Starbuck *et al.*, 2011); b) monitor the effect of changes in technique and shoe–surface combination on lower limb geometry, sliding and forces underfoot (Stiles and Dixon, 2006; Damm *et al.*, 2011); c) monitor the effect of human movement on surface wear, degradation and performance properties (Stiles *et al.*, 2009; Guisasola *et al.*, 2010); and d) continue monitoring injury incidence as shoes and surfaces develop.

## Key summary points

- There is some evidence that surface characteristics which influence cushioning and/or friction can have an effect on the risk of injury when performing on the surface. However, conclusive statements regarding mechanical characteristics and the influence on injury risk cannot be made.
- Surface characteristics influencing cushioning and/or friction result in measurable changes in lower limb biomechanics. Surfaces with low cushioning have been observed to increase loading at the shoe–surface interface. Similarly, high shoe–surface friction can cause relatively high loading.
- There is evidence that changes in specific biomechanical variables, including peak loading rates, pressure patterns under the foot and joint moments, are related to the development of injury.
- Studies which simultaneously quantify surface characteristics, injury incidence and biomechanics are required to strengthen our understanding of the role of sports surfaces in influencing injury risk.
- Compared to running, analysis of sport-specific movements are most suitable for detecting biomechanical differences with changes in traction and hardness properties of surfaces.
- Perception influences player attitudes to changes in surface which may have a bearing on player–shoe–surface interaction and sports surface development to optimise performance and minimise injury risk.

## References

Andersson, H., Ekblom, B. and Krustrup, P. (2008) 'Elite football on synthetic turf versus natural grass: Movement patterns, technical standards, and player impressions', *Journal of Sports Sciences,* 26: 113–122.

Andreasson, G. and Olofsson, B. (1983) 'Surface and shoe deformation in sport activities and injuries', in B. M. Nigg and B. A. Kerr (eds) *The Biomechanical Aspects of Sport Shoes and Playing Surfaces*. Canada: University of Calgary.

Bastholt, P. (2000) 'Professional tennis (ATP Tour) and number of medical treatments in relation to type of surface', *Medicine and Science in Tennis,* 5.

BBC Sport (2012) 'Novak Djokovic irritated by Madrid Open blue clay'. Available at: www.bbc.co.uk/sport/0/tennis/18000107 (accessed 9 May 2012).

Bennell, K., Crossley, K., Jayarajan, J., Walton, E., Warden, S., Kiss, Z. S. and Wrigley, T. (2004) 'Ground reaction forces and bone parameters in females with tibial stress fracture', *Medicine and Science in Sports and Exercise,* 6: 397–404.

Bennell, K., Creaby, M. W., Wrigley, T. V., Bowles, K., Hinman, R., Cicuttini, F. and Hunter, D. J. (2010) 'Bone marrow lesions are related to dynamic knee loading in medial knee osteoarthritis', *Annals of the Rheumatic Diseases*, 69: 1151–1154.Annals of the Rheumatic Disease 69: 1151-1154.

Beukeboom, C., Birmingham, T. B., Forwell, L. and Ohrling, D. (2000) 'Asymmetrical strength changes and injuries in athletes training on a small radius curve indoor track', *Clinical Journal of Sports Medicine*, 10: 245–250.

Bjørneboe, J., Bahr, R. and Andersen, T. E. (2010) 'Risk of injury on third-generation synthetic turf in Norwegian professional football', *British Journal of Sports Medicine*, 44: 794–798.

Bobbert, M. F., Yeadon, M. R. and Nigg, B. M. (1992) 'Mechanical analysis of the landing phase in heel-toe running', *Journal of Biomechanics*, 25: 223–234.

Bowers, K. D. Jr and Martin, R. B. (1974) 'Impact absorption, new and old AstroTurf at West Virginia University', *Medicine and Science in Sports*, 6: 217–221.

Brito, J., Krustrup, P. and Rebelo, A. (2012) 'The influence of the playing surface on the exercise intensity of small-sided recreational soccer games', *Human Movement Science*, 31: 946–956.

Canaway, P. M., Bell, M. J., Holmes, G. and Baker S. W. (1990) 'Standards for the playing quality of natural turf for association football', in R. C. Schmidt., E. F. Hoerner, E. N. Milner and C. A. Morehouse (eds) *Natural and Artificial Playing Fields: Characteristics and Safety Features*. Phoenix, Arizona; Philadelphia: ASTM.

Clarke, T. E., Frederick, E. C. and Cooper, L. B. (1983a) 'Biomechanical measurement of running shoe cushioning properties', in B. M. Nigg and B. A. Kerr (eds) *The Biomechanical Aspects of Sport Shoes and Playing Surfaces*. Canada: University of Calgary.

Clarke, T. E., Frederick, E. C. and Cooper, L. B. (1983b) 'Effects of cushioning upon ground reaction forces in running', *International Journal of Sports Medicine*, 4: 247–251.

Clement, D. B. Taunton, J. E. and Smart, G. W. (1984) 'Achilles tendinitis and peritendinitis: Etiology and treatment', *American Journal of Sports Medicine*, 12: 179–184.

Coren, S., Porac, C. and Ward, L. M. (1979) *Sensation and Perception*. London: Academic Press.

Cross, R. (2006) 'Grand Slam injuries 1978–2005', *Medicine and Science in Tennis*, 11:1.

Crossley, K., Bennell, K. L., Wrigley, T. and Oakes, B. W. (1999) 'Ground reaction forces, bone characteristics, and tibial stress fracture in male runners', *Medicine and Science in Sports and Exercise*, 31(8): 1088–1093.

Damm, L., Low, D., Richardson, A., Clarke, J., Carré, M. and Dixon, S. D. (2011) 'Modulation of tennis players' frictional demand according to surface traction characteristics', Paper presented at International Society of Biomechanics Congress XXIII, Brussels, Belgium, July 2011.

De Wit, B. and De Clercq, D. (1997) 'Differences in sagittal plane kinematics between barefoot and shod running', Paper presented at the Second Annual Congress of the European College of Sports Sciences, Copenhagen, Denmark, August 1997.

De Wit, B., De Clercq, D. and Aerts, P. (2000) 'Biomechanical analysis of the stance phase during barefoot and shod running', *Journal of Biomechanics*, 33: 269–278.

Dick, R. W., Schmalz, R., Diehl, N., Newlin, C. and Summers, E. (2003) 'A review of game injuries by surface and injury mechanism in NCAA intercollegiate sports', in B. M. Nigg, G. K. Cole and D. J. Stefanyshyn (eds) *Sports Surfaces*. Canada: University of Calgary.

Dixon, S. J. and Stiles, V. H. (2003) 'Impact absorption of tennis shoe-surface combinations', *Sports Engineering*, 6: 1–9.

Dixon, S. J., Batt, M. E., Collop, A. C. and Singleton, T. M. (1998) 'The biomechanical and mechanical performance of Sureflexâ sports surface material', in S. J. Haake (ed.) *The Engineering of Sport*. Cambridge: Blackwell Science.

Dixon, S. J., Collop, A. C. and Batt, M. E. (2000) 'Surface effects on ground reaction forces and lower extremity kinematics in running', *Medicine and Science in Sports Exercise*, 32: 1919–1926.

Dowling, A. V., Corazza, S., Chaudhari, A.M.W. and Andriacchi, T. P. (2010) 'Shoe-surface friction influences movement strategies during a sidestep cutting task', *The American Journal of Sports Medicine*, 38: 478–485.

Dragoo, J. L. and Braun, H. J. (2010) 'The effect of playing surface on injury rate: A review of the current literature', *Sports Medicine*, 40: 981–990.

Ekstrand, J. and Nigg, B. M. (1989) 'Surface-related injuries in soccer', *Sports Medicine*, 8: 56–62.

Ekstrand, J., Hägglund, M. and Fuller, C. W. (2011) 'Comparison of injuries sustained on synthetic turf and grass by male and female elite football players', *Scandinavian Journal of Medicine and Science in Sports*, 21: 824–832.

Fleming, P. R., Young, C., Roberts, J. R., Jones, R. and Dixon, N. (2005) 'Human perceptions of synthetic surfaces for field hockey', *Sports Engineering*, 8: 121–136.

Ford, K. R., Manson, N. A., Evans, B. J., Myer, G. D., Gwin, R. C., Heidt, R. S. Jr and Hewett, T. E. (2006) 'Comparison of in-shoe loading patterns on natural grass and synthetic turf', *Journal of Science and Medicine in Sport*, 9: 433–440.

Fuller, C. W., Dick, R. W., Corlette, J. and Schmalz, R. (2007a) 'Comparison of the incidence, nature and cause of injuries sustained on grass and new generation synthetic turf by male and female football players. Part 1: match injuries', *British Journal of Sports Medicine*, 41: SI i20–i26.

Fuller, C.W., Dick, R.W., Corlette, J. and Schmalz, R. (2007b) 'Comparison of the incidence, nature and cause of injuries sustained on grass and new generation synthetic turf by male and female football players. Part 2: training injuries', *British Journal of Sports Medicine*, 41: SI i27–i32.

Girard, O., Eicher, F., Fourchet, F., Micallef, J. P. and Millet, G. P. (2007) 'Effects of the playing surface on plantar pressures and potential injuries in tennis', *British Journal of Sports Medicine*, 41: 733–738.

Griffin, L. Y., Albohm, M. J., Arendt, E. A., Bahr, R., Beynnon, B. D., DeMaio, M., Dick, R. W., Engebretsen, L., Garrett, W. E., Hannafin, J. A., Hewitt, T. E., Huston, L. J., Ireland, M. L., Johnson, R. J., Lephart, S., Mandelbaum, B. R., Mann, B. J., Marks, P. H., Marshall, S. W., Myklebust, G., Noyes, F. R., Powers, C., Shields Jr, C., Shultz, S. J., Silvers, H., Slauterbeck, J., Taylor, D. C., Teitz, C. C., Wojtys, E. M. and Yu, B. (2006) 'Understanding and preventing noncontact anterior cruciate ligament injuries', *The American Journal of Sports Medicine*, 34: 1512–1532.

Grimston, S. K., Engsberg, J. R., Kloiber, R. and Hanley, D. A. (1991) 'Bone mass, external loads, and stress fractures in female runners', *International Journal of Sport Biomechanics*, 7: 293–302.

Guisasola, I., James, I., Stiles, V. and Dixon, S. (2010) 'Dynamic behaviour of soils used for natural turf sports surfaces', *Sports Engineering*, 12: 111–122.

Hamill, J., van Emmerik, R.E.A. and Heiderscheit, B. C. (1999) 'A dynamical systems approach to lower extremity running injuries', *Clinical Biomechanics*, 14: 297–308.

Hennig, E. M., Valiant, G. A. and Liu, Q. (1996) 'Biomechanical variables and the perception of cushioning for running in various types of footwear', *Journal of Applied Biomechanics*, 12: 143–150.

Hodgson-Phillips, L. (2000) 'Sports injury incidence', *British Journal of Sports Medicine*, 34: 133–136.

Hreljac, A., Marshall, R. N. and Hume, P. A. (2000) 'Evaluation of lower extremity overuse injury potential in runners', *Medicine and Science in Sports and Exercise*, 32: 1635–1641.

James, S. L., Bates, B. T. and Osternig, L. R. (1978) 'Injuries to runners', *The American Journal of Sports Medicine*, 6: 40–50.

Keene, J. S., Narechania, R. G., Sachtjen, K. M. and Clancy, W. G. (1980) 'Tartan Turf® on trial', *The American Journal of Sports Medicine*, 8: 43–47.

Kulund, D. N., McCue, F. C. 3rd, Rockwell, D. A. and Gieck, J. H. (1979) 'Tennis injuries: prevention and treatment: A review', *The American Journal of Sports Medicine*, 7: 249–253.

Larson, R. L. and Osternig, L. R. (1974) 'Traumatic bursitis and synthetic turf', *Journal of Sports Medicine*, 2: 183–188.

Lilley, K., Dixon, S. and Stiles, V. (2011) 'A biomechanical comparison of the running gait of mature and young females', *Gait and Posture*, 33: 496–500.

Lynch, S. A. and Renström, A.F.H. (2002) 'Lower leg and Achilles tendon problems in tennis', in P.A.F.H. Renström (ed.) *Tennis*. Oxford: Blackwell Publishing.

Martinez, A., Dura, J. V., Duenas, L, Gámez, J., Alemany, S. and González, J. C. (2004) 'Synthetic and natural turf: biomechanical differences between surfaces', *Journal of Sports Science*, 22: 494–495.

McCarthy, P. (1989) 'Synthetic turf: Does it cause more injuries?', *Physician and Sports Medicine*, 17: 159–164.

Messier, S. P., Edwards, D. G., Martin, D. F., Lowery, R. B., Canon, D. W., James, M. K., Curl, W. W., Read, H. M. and Hunter, D. M. (1995) 'Etiology of iliotibial band friction syndrome in distance runners', *Medicine and Science in Sports and Exercise*, 27, 951–960.

Milburn, P. D. and Barry, E. B. (1998) 'Shoe–surface interaction and the reduction of injury in rugby union', *Journal of Sports Medicine*, 25: 319–327.

Miller, S. (2006) 'Modern tennis rackets, balls, and surfaces', *British Journal of Sports Medicine*, 40: 401–405.

Milner, C. E., Ferber, R., Pollard, C. D., Hamill, J. and Davis, I. S. (2006) 'Biomechanical factors associated with tibial stress fracture in female runners', *Medicine and Science in Sports and Exercise*, 38: 323–328.

Miyazaki, T., Wada, M., Kawahara, H., Sato, M., Baba, H. and Shimada, S. (2002) 'Dynamic load at baseline can predict radiographic disease progression in medial compartment knee osteoarthritis', *Annals of the Rheumatic Diseases*, 61: 617–622.

Nigg, B. M. (1983) 'External force measurements with sport shoes and playing surfaces', in B. M. Nigg and B. A. Kerr (eds) *Biomechanical Aspects of Sport Shoes and Playing Surfaces*. Calgary: University Printing.

Nigg, B. M. and Segesser, B. (1988) 'The influence of playing surfaces on the load on the locomotor system and on football and tennis injuries', *Sports Medicine*, 5: 375–385.

Nigg, B. M. and Yeadon, M. R. (1987) 'Biomechanical aspects of playing surfaces', *Journal of Sports Science*, 5: 117–145.

Nigg, B. M., Frederick, E. C., Hawes, M. R. and Luethi, S. M. (1986) 'Factors influencing short-term pain and injuries in tennis', *Journal of Applied Biomechanics*, 2: 156–165.

Nigg, B. M., Stefanyshyn, D. J., Rozitis, A. I. and Mundermann, A. (2009) 'Resultant knee joint moments for lateral movement tasks on sliding and non-sliding sport surfaces', *Journal of Sports Sciences*, 27(5): 427–435.

Norton, K., Schwerdt, S. and Lange, K. (2001) 'Evidence for the aetiology of injury in Australian football', *British Journal of Sports Medicine*, 35: 418–423.

Nunns, M. (2014) *Biomechanical Predictors of Tibial and Third Metatarsal Stress Fractures in Royal Marine Recruits*, unpublished PhD thesis, University of Exeter, UK.

Olsen, O. E., Myklebust, G., Engebretsen, L., Holme, I. and Bahr, R. (2003) 'Relationship between floor type and risk of ACL injury in team handball', *Scandinavian Journal of Medicine and Science in Sports*, 13: 299–304.

Orchard, J. (2001) 'The AFL Penetrometer study: Work in progress', *Journal of Science and Medicine in Sport*, 4: 220–232.

Orchard, J. (2002) 'Is there a relationship between ground and climatic conditions and injuries in football?', *Journal of Sports Medicine*, 32: 419–432.

Orchard, J., Chivers, I. H., Aldous, D. E., Bennell, K. and Seward, H. (2005) 'Rye grass is associated with fewer non-contact anterior cruciate ligament injuries than Bermuda grass', *British Journal of Sports Medicine*, 39: 704–709.

Orchard, J., Rodas, G., Til, L., Ardevòl, J. and Chivers, I. (2008) 'A hypothesis: Could portable natural grass be a risk factor for knee injuries?', *Journal of Sports Science and Medicine*, 7: 184–190.

Powell, J. W. and Schootman, M. (1992) 'A multivariate risk analysis of selected playing surfaces in the National Football League: 1980–1989. An epidemiologic study of knee injuries', *The American Journal of Sports Medicine*, 20: 686–694.

Radin, E. L., Yang, K. H., Reigger, C., Kish, V. L. and O'Connor J. J. (1991) 'Relationship between lower limb dynamics and knee joint pain', *Journal of Orthopedic Research*, 9: 398–405.

Renström, P.A.F.H. and Lynch, S. A. (2002) 'Knee injuries in tennis', in P.A.F.H. Renström (ed.) *Tennis*. Oxford: Blackwell Publishing.

Rice, H., Nunns, M., House, C., Fallowfield, J., Allsopp, A. and Dixon, S. (2013) 'High medial plantar pressures during barefoot running are associated with increased risk of ankle inversion injury in Royal Marine recruits', *Gait Posture*, 38(4): 614–618.

Rogers III, J. N. and Waddington, D. V. (1990) 'Effects of management practices on impact absorption and shear resistance in natural turf', in R. C. Schmidt, E. F. Hoerner, E. N. Milner and C. A. Morehouse (eds) *Natural and Artificial*

*Playing Fields: Characteristics and Safety Features*. Phoenix, Arizona; Philadelphia: ASTM.

Shorten, M. R. (2000) 'Running shoe design: Protection and performance', in D. Tunstall Pedoe (ed.) *Marathon Medicine*. London: Royal Society of Medicine.

Soligard, T., Bahr, R. and Andersen, T. E. (2012) 'Injury risk on synthetic turf and grass in youth tournament football', *Scandinavian Journal of Medicine and Science in Sports*, 22: 356–361.

Starbuck, C., Stiles, V., Miller, S. and Dixon, S. (2011) 'Player perceptions of tennis surfaces', Paper presented at the BASES Biomechanics Interest Group Easter Meeting, University of Chichester, April 2011.

Starbuck, C. (2015) *Biomechanics and Player Perceptions of Tennis Surfaces*, unpublished PhD thesis, University of Exeter, UK.

Stefanyshyn, D., Stergiou, P., Lun, V.M.Y., Meeuwisse, W. H. and Worobets, J. T. (2006) 'Knee angular impulse as a predictor of patellofemoral pain in runners', *American Journal of Sports Medicine*, 34: 1844–1851.

Steffen, K., Andersen, T. E. and Bahr, R. (2007) 'Risk of injury on synthetic turf and natural grass in young female football players', *British Journal of Sports Medicine*, 41: SI i33–i37.

Stiles, V. H. and Dixon, S. J. (2006) 'The influence of different playing surfaces on the biomechanics of a tennis running forehand foot plant', *Journal of Applied Biomechanics*, 22: 14–24.

Stiles, V. H. and Dixon, S. J. (2007) 'Biomechanical response to systematic changes in impact interface cushioning properties while performing a tennis specific movement', *Journal of Sports Sciences*, 25: 1229–1239.

Stiles, V. H., James, I. T., Dixon, S. J. and Guisasola, I. N. (2009) 'Natural turf surfaces: The case for continued research', *Sports Medicine*, 39: 65–84.

Stiles, V. H., Guisasola, I. N., James, I. T. and Dixon, S. J. (2011) 'Biomechanical response to changes in natural turf during running and turning', *Journal of Applied Biomechanics*, 27: 54–63.

Stucke, H., Baudzus, W. and Baumann, W. (1984) 'On friction characteristics of playing surfaces', in F. C. Frederick (ed.) *Sports Shoes and Playing Surfaces*. Champaign, IL: Human Kinetics.

Taunton, J. E., Ryan, M. B., Clement, D. B., McKenzie, D. C., Lloyd-Smith, D. R. and Zumbo, B. D. (2003) 'A prospective study of running injuries: The Vancouver Sun Run "in training" clinics', *British Journal of Sports Medicine*, 37: 239–244.

Torg, J., Quendenfeld, T. and Landau, B. (1974) 'The shoe-surface interface and its relationship to football knee injuries', *Journal of Sports Medicine*, 2: 261–269.

Visell, Y., Giordano, B. L., Millet, G. and Cooperstock, J. R. (2011) 'Vibration influences haptic perception of surface compliance during walking', *PLoS ONE*, 6: e17697.

Wang, L., Hong, Y., Li, J. X. and Zhou, J. H. (2012) 'Comparison of plantar loads during running on different overground surfaces', *Research in Sports Medicine*, 20: 75–85.

Willems, T. M., Witvrouw, E., Delbaere, K., De Cock, A. and De Clercq, D. (2005) 'Relationship between gait biomechanics and inversion sprains: A prospective study of risk factors', *Gait and Posture*, 21(4): 379–387.

Willems, T. M., Witvrouw, E., De Cock, A. and De Clercq, D. (2007) 'Gait-related risk factors for exercise-related lower-leg pain during shod running', *Medicine and Science in Sports and Exercise*, 39(2): 330–339.

Williams, S., Hume, P. A. and Kara, S. (2011) 'A review of football injuries on third and fourth generation synthetic turfs compared with natural turf', *Sports Medicine*, 41: 903–923.

Yu, B. and Garrett, W. E. (2007) 'Mechanisms of non-contact ACL injuries', *British Journal of Sports Medicine*, 41: S1 i47–i51.

Yu, B., Lin, C-F. and Garrett, W. E. (2006) 'Lower extremity biomechanics during the landing of a stop-jump task', *Clinical Biomechanics*, 21: 297–305.

Chapter 5

# Sports surfaces and performance

*Darren Stefanyshyn and John Wannop*

## Introduction

It is well-known that sports surfaces can have a considerable effect on performance. This chapter focuses on the influence that sports surfaces have on performance through the interaction with the athlete. In general there are two main sports surface characteristics that have been linked with an athlete's performance: a) surface traction and b) cushioning or compliance of the surface.

Traction between the shoe and surface has long been known to influence sports performance. If a surface does not provide sufficient traction, an athlete will slip and performance will be compromised. However, it is only recently that the relationship between traction and performance has been studied scientifically. These recent studies will be explored in this chapter.

Traditionally, when considering the influence of cushioning on sports performance, the concept of energy storage and return is discussed. This concept will be examined in this chapter. It is also becoming apparent that surface compliance can influence how an athlete's muscles generate force and work, which directly influences performance. This aspect will also be discussed.

## Surface traction

Traction between the surface and shoe is one of the most important aspects of design in relation to performance. In fact, soccer athletes rate traction as the second most desirable shoe property next only to comfort (Sterzing *et al.*, 2007). Traction takes place at the interface between the shoe and surface, affecting the ability of the athlete to generate forces which enable the athlete to accelerate, decelerate and perform rapid changes in direction (Fleming, 2011).

A recent study examining the effects of traction on performance determined that modifications of traction of only 20 percent can have large effects on performance (Worobets and Wannop, 2012). Athletes executed three movements while wearing different shoes; a vertical jump, a short sprint and an agility cutting course. The results of the study revealed that a reduction of traction of 20 percent resulted in a significant reduction in performance of all three tasks while increases in traction of 20 percent resulted in significant increases in performance of the vertical jump and the agility cutting course.

The results of the study seem to follow the general belief that maximizing the amount of traction will maximise the athlete's performance. One important aspect that is often not considered, however, has to do with the relationship between the maximum available traction and the traction which the athlete can actually utilise. The maximum available traction is the maximum traction that can be used, usually quantified using simple mechanical traction tests. This value is different to the utilised traction by the athlete, which represents the actual amount of traction that the athlete uses during a specific athletic movement. Simply because a specific shoe–surface combination is able to attain a high traction value during mechanical testing, does not mean that the athlete will use all the traction that the shoe is able to provide during the athletic task.

A study examining the balance between the maximum available traction and the actual utilised traction was recently published (Luo and Stefanyshyn, 2011). Athletes performed curve sprinting movements while wearing shoes with different amounts of maximum available traction (measured during a mechanical drag test). The results showed that athletes used all of the mechanically available traction while wearing the shoes with low traction; however the athletes seemed to generally utilise the same amount of available traction while wearing the mid and high traction shoes (Figure 5.1a). Only at the start and end, for very short periods of time during ground contact, did the athletes make use of the higher available traction. This result indicates that there is a certain threshold of available traction that athletes can utilise during specific athletic movements. Even if the maximum available traction is much greater than this threshold, athletes did not utilise the traction above this threshold. The performance results of the test were similar to the traction results, as there were increases in performance of a curved sprint going from low to mid traction shoes, but no increases in performance when athletes went from the mid to the high traction shoes (Figure 5.1b). This study clearly demonstrates that increasing traction does increase performance, but only to a certain critical point, which is dictated by the average utilised traction. Increasing available traction values above this threshold does not influence performance due to the fact that the athletes cannot utilise any more of the available traction.

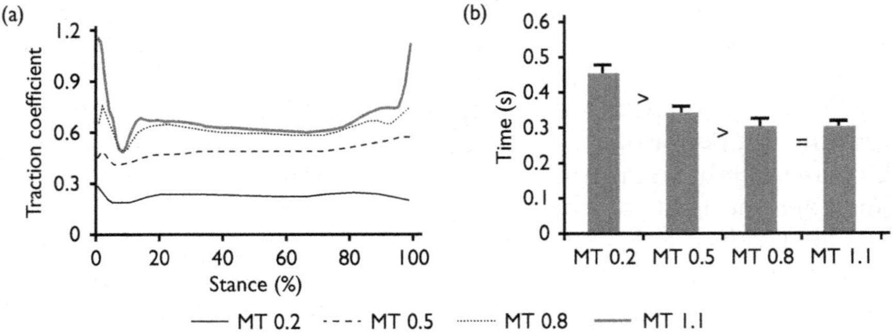


*Figure 5.1* (a) The traction coefficient of four shoes with different amounts of maximum available traction: measured traction (MT) values of 0.2, 0.5, 0.8 and 1.1. The curves represent the average of all subjects and are normalised to stance time of the athletes performing a circular sprint test (fine black curve=MT0.2, dashed curve=MT0.5, dotted curve=MT0.8 and solid grey curve=MT1.1); (b) average performance results of the four shoes with different amounts of maximum available traction. The values represent the average circular sprint time to cover a distance of 1m for all subjects in each condition.

Alterations to the traction at the shoe–surface interface can influence performance, however simply maximizing the amount of available traction will not continually increase an athlete's performance, and may in fact induce some negative effects on the athlete. Chapter 4 highlighted how increases in traction may be detrimental in terms of athlete safety, leading to increases in injury risk. This introduces the concept of optimal traction, with an intricate balance of adequate traction to maximise performance while keeping traction low enough to prevent an increase in injury risk.

It is clear that alterations in traction can affect performance, but the studies presented thus far have primarily examined changes in footwear properties to modify traction. Since traction is influenced by both the shoe and surface, alterations in the surface will also result in traction changes and, therefore, could have potential for altering performance. A wealth of studies have compared the maximum available traction of different surfaces using pure mechanical tests (Bonstingl *et al.*, 1975; Lambson *et al.*, 1996; Livesay *et al.*, 2006; Stanitski *et al.*, 1974; Torg *et al.*, 1974; Villwock *et al.*, 2009b; Wannop and Stefanyshyn, 2012; Worobets and Wannop, 2012). The results of these studies indicate that small to substantial changes in traction can occur by changing the playing surface (the magnitude of traction changes depends on the extent of the surface change as well as testing methods).

Large changes in traction occur on different turf surfaces, with traction values increasing as much as 30 percent for an infill artificial turf compared to a native soil-based natural grass surface (Villwock *et al.*, 2009a). However, performance results comparing natural grass and artificial turf are sparse, with the few studies presenting conflicting results. Some studies found increases in performance on artificial turf (Gains *et al.*, 2010; Potthast, 2010); however, other studies showed no performance differences between the two surfaces (Ford *et al.*, 2006). Traction differences of over 20 percent should enable changes in performance (Worobets and Wannop, 2012), however, a lack of traction testing in these performance studies has limited the interpretation of the results. It could be that in the studies with no difference in performance, there were only small differences in traction between the surfaces. In addition it is possible that the athletes had already reached their peak utilised traction while on the grass surface; therefore, even though the artificial surface increased the amount of available traction, the athletes did not utilise any of this increase.

There is a multitude of different artificial turf surfaces currently being utilised for sport, with surfaces encompassing different fibre types, fibre lengths and types of infill material depending on the specific sport and environment they are to be utilised for. Research has shown that each of these variables can have an influence on the traction of the surface. Polyethylene fibers have been shown to produce lower traction than nylon fiber carpets (approximately 6 percent lower), likely due to the softer yarn (Young, 2006). Cryogenic rubber infill material has been shown to provide higher traction (approximately 10 percent higher) when compared to crumb rubber infill (Villwock *et al.*, 2009b). Increases in the compaction or bulk density of the infill material leads to the general trend of increasing traction (with differences in traction values of up to 10 percent) (Severn *et al.*, 2011). The age of the surface can also affect the traction values, with older surfaces having traction increases of approximately 15 percent (Severn *et al.*, 2010).

Studies thoroughly investigating whether any of these aspects affecting surface traction can have a significant influence on performance are limited. One study has shown performance differences on two types of artificial turf surfaces (Potthast *et al.*, 2010), with performance being defined as ball-kicking accuracy. Unfortunately the characteristics of the surfaces were not clearly identified other than the fact that one consisted of an all-rubber infill, while the other consisted of a sand and rubber infill. The results showed that kicking accuracy was lower on the sand and rubber infill compared to the all-rubber infill surface. The change in infill material altered the kinematics of the movement of the athlete, which in turn influenced the kicking performance. Another study examined the effect that a standard SBR (Styrene-butadiene rubber) infill and a TPE (Thermoplastic elastomere) infill had on the kinematics and kinetics during a sprint start. The SBR surface had higher translational traction and during testing it was found that athletes could develop a much larger horizontal impulse on the SBR surface, which could lead to an increase in performance (Potthast *et al.*, 2010; Verhelst, 2010).

A multitude of factors of the sport surface can affect traction but not many studies have detailed the effects these factors can have on performance. Of the studies that have been conducted, the definition and description of the surfaces used during testing was often lacking. As well, differences between in-lab testing on sample surfaces and on-field testing (Severn *et al.*, 2011) can further cloud the results and conclusions reached. Overall, however, it appears that increases in surface traction can increase performance, but only up to a certain critical point.

### *Surface cushioning – compliance*

As an athlete lands and contacts the surface, energy is transferred from the athlete to the surface and is stored in the surface as potential energy. When the athlete leaves the surface, some of this deformation energy can return from the surface to the athlete. The magnitude of the energy returned from a sport surface can have a large influence on athletic performance and is directly related to the amount of energy input into the surface minus the energy lost.

The energy input into a surface is a function of the force the athlete exerts on the surface during ground contact. Sporting movements are associated with large forces. For example, intense activities like landing from a jump can generate ground contact forces of over 8000N and even relatively simple movements like jogging can produce peak contact forces of 2000N (Nigg, 1999). These large forces that athletes exert on sports surfaces provide the energy to compress the surface and allow for deformation energy to be stored. The actual magnitude of the stored energy depends on the properties of the surface such as surface stiffness. The more compliant the surface, the larger the deformation and the greater the energy stored.

The stiffness of very compliant surfaces like tumbling floors and gymnastics surfaces have been reported to be approximately 50–100kN/m (Stefanyshyn and Nigg, 2000). When loaded by a gymnast, the compliant floors deform 5–10cm and from a performance perspective allow a gymnast to increase jump height by about 0.2m and flight time by about 0.2s, allowing more time to perform complex aerial maneuvers (Stefanyshyn and Nigg, 2000).

The previous example assumed the gymnastics floor acts like an ideal linear spring where all of the energy stored in the surface is returned to the gymnast. However, not all of the energy will be returned as some of the energy will be lost to aspects such as heat, sound and vibrations that do not benefit the athlete's performance. Thus, in returning to its original shape, the work done by the surface on the athlete is less than the work done by the athlete to deform the surface. This dissipated energy is a material property that is common to all surfaces and cannot be avoided. However, the magnitude of the energy dissipation can be influenced.

Energy loss varies widely between different types of surfaces. In a sample experiment, drop tests with varying inputs (different masses dropped from different heights) were performed on infilled turf and point elastic surfaces (Figure 5.2). The majority of the energy input into the infilled surface was lost (about 85 percent). The sand/rubber mixture in the infilled turf is designed primarily to cushion landings and is not well-suited to store and return energy. The point elastic track surfaces had substantially greater energy return than the infilled surfaces. Within the group of point elastic surfaces, there were substantial differences in energy return, despite the fact that all the surfaces were constructed for installation as a competitive running track.

Data from mechanical drop tests used to quantify energy loss of a sports surface must be interpreted with caution as they often don't correlate well with subject tests and they may overestimate the energy lost during actual sport activities (Nigg and Yeadon, 1987). It has been suggested that the short contact times during mechanical impacts, which happen much quicker than a typical ground contact of an athlete, are not indicative as they do not provide sufficient time for the surface to expand to its original thickness. Using a finite element model, it has been estimated the energy loss in a typical running surface is only 1–2 percent when

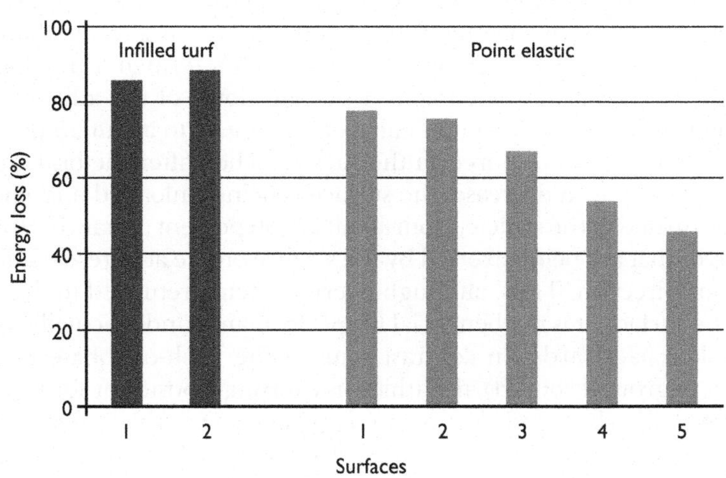


*Figure 5.2* Average results of energy loss values for two infilled turf and five point elastic surfaces as measured from vertical drop tests using two spherical masses from three different heights.

actual ground reaction forces measured during running were used as inputs (Baroud *et al.*, 1999a).

Even using a very conservative estimate of only 50 percent of the energy that is input into a typical sports surface being returned (energy loss of 50 percent) this magnitude is substantial enough to influence athletic performance. For example, it has been estimated that the total mechanical energy required for a running stride is somewhere around 100–200J (Ker *et al.*, 1987; Baroud *et al.*, 1999b). Furthermore, it has been estimated that running tracks deform about 1cm and store approximately 12J of energy during a typical sprinting stride (Stefanyshyn and Nigg, 2000). Energy return of 6J would represent over 3 percent of the mechanical energy per stride. If all of this returned energy aids performance, a 3 percent increase in performance relates to about 0.3 seconds in an elite-level 100m race. This description is an oversimplification and it is unlikely that all of the returned energy goes directly into athletic performance, however it demonstrates the importance of energy return from sports surfaces.

Energy is a scalar quantity and, therefore, energy return is independent of direction. However, the forces exerted by a surface as energy are returned to an athlete as vector quantities, having both magnitude and direction. Therefore, for an athlete to make effective use of the returned energy, the forces from the surface must be exerted in the proper direction.

To understand the importance of directionality of forces during energy return it is helpful to consider the anterior-posterior ground reaction force during running (Figure 5.3). During the landing phase the athlete is exerting an anteriorly directed force on the surface. As a result, the surface is exerting a posterior force on the athlete, often termed a braking force since the net result of this force is a slowing down of the athlete. As this braking force increases, from initial ground contact to about 25 percent of stance, energy is being stored in the surface. Then after the braking force peaks and begins to decrease, the surface is being unloaded and energy is being returned to the athlete, from about 25–50 percent of stance. However, the forces that are being exerted by the surface on the athlete are still in the posterior direction. Thus, although energy is being returned to the athlete from the surface, it is not beneficial for performance and is actually pushing the athlete backwards. In contrast, during the push-off phase (latter 50 percent of ground contact), the athlete is exerting a posterior force pushing back on the surface and the surface is pushing the athlete forward. As a result, the energy stored in the surface from about 50–75 percent of stance can be returned to the athlete during the last 25 percent of stance. The direction that the surface exerts force is important for appropriately utilizing the stored energy and it has been shown that modifying the directionality of structural elements in a surface can have a large influence on the magnitude of energy returned to an athlete (Baroud *et al.*, 1999b).

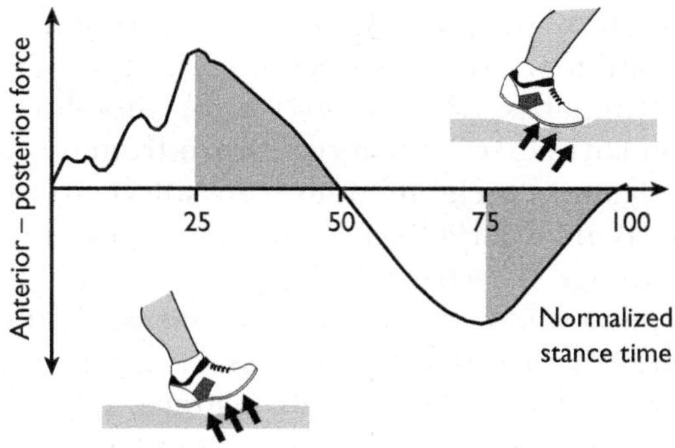


*Figure 5.3* Ground reaction force in the anterior-posterior direction during running demonstrating the directionality of the force applied on the athlete. The shaded regions indicate times of energy return from the surface to the athlete.

In addition to directionality, it has been proposed that energy return should occur with the right frequency, at the appropriate time and at the right location (Nigg and Segesser, 1992). It is important to match the frequency of the surface to the rate of loading and unloading of the activity. For example, sprinters contact the surface for about 100ms. Since the deformation and release correspond roughly to one-half of a sinus wave, one full cycle then corresponds to 200ms, or a frequency of 5Hz. Optimal sprinting surfaces should, therefore, try to match this loading and unloading frequency of around 5Hz (Stafilidis and Arampatzis, 2007). The appropriate time and location for energy return is when the athlete is in the right position to utilise the energy return, that is during takeoff. For the running example presented in Figure 5.3, the energy return in the first half of stance is at the wrong location and not at the right time, it is being returned too early, before the athlete is in the right position to benefit from the energy return.

It is clear that the storage and return of mechanical energy in a compliant surface can influence performance. However, it is important to realise that when considering the interaction between an athlete and a sports surface one must also take the athlete into account, not just the surface. That is, the system as a whole is biomechanical not just mechanical, and while the material properties of the surface determine its behavior, an athlete can change his or her biomechanical properties when interacting with different surfaces (Arampatzis *et al.*, 2001; Hardin *et al.*, 2004). For example as surface stiffness increases athletes land with more extended legs and have greater peak angular velocities of their ankle, knee and hip joints.

The musculoskeletal system is a complex combination of muscles, tendons and ligaments. Muscle force generation is dependent on intrinsic characteristics such as muscle length and contraction velocity. Surface compliance can influence the force generation of muscles (Sanders and Allen, 1993; Arampatzis *et al.*, 2004) and, therefore, performance. Additionally, similar to external energy return from the surface, internal energy return from muscle tendons can affect sports performance (Alexander and Bennett, 1989) and surface compliance can influence tendon energy storage (Bosco *et al.*, 1997).

When performing submaximal activities such as running, jumping and hopping on surfaces of different stiffness, it is difficult to notice any difference in the athlete's movement pattern. The centre of mass displacement is kept constant as are parameters such as stride frequency, ground contact time and peak ground reaction forces (Farley *et al.*, 1998; Ferris *et al.*, 1998, 1999). It appears that athletes regulate these variables independent of surface stiffness but to do this they must be changing their internal muscle-tendon characteristics. The net result is a change in the athlete's leg stiffness and it has been shown that as surface stiffness increases, leg stiffness decreases such that the combined stiffness of the two "springs" in series remains fairly constant (Farley *et al.*, 1998; Ferris *et al.*, 1998; Moritz and Farley, 2005). For hopping the leg stiffness is primarily regulated at the ankle joint (Ferris and Farley, 1997) while regulation occurs primarily at the knee during running (Arampatzis *et al.*, 1999).

When combined with the mechanical energy returned from the surface, the biomechanical changes resulting from changes in surface stiffness can be optimised to maximise performance. Studies on track surfaces with different compliance (McMahon and Greene, 1978, 1979) showed that there is an optimal stiffness that maximises performance. McMahon and Greene developed a theoretical model that predicted that the athletes would be fastest on an infinitely stiff surface without any deformation, a theory that has also been proposed by others (Stafilidis and Arampatzis, 2007). However, this was only true if the runner was modelled as an ideal elastic system without any damping, which is unrealistic. When the runner was modeled with internal damping and energy dissipation their model suggested an intermediate stiffness would maximise the energy return and running speed. This optimal stiffness was determined to be approximately 2–4 times the lower leg stiffness (160–320 kN/m) and the model predicted a 1–3 percent increase in running speed at these stiffnesses. Harvard University built a new running track based on these results, with a stiffness of approximately 240kN/m. Experimental results on this track verified the model predictions as speed enhancements of approximately 2 percent were realised. Other theoretical models have predicted similar results, namely that work performed by a runner can be minimised by providing an optimal surface stiffness (Nigg and Anton, 1995).

Other experimental studies have also shown direct influences on performance due to surface compliance. For example, running becomes more economical as surface stiffness decreases. The metabolic cost of running, as measured by oxygen consumption, was found to decrease by 12 percent when surface stiffness was decreased from 945.7kN/m to 75.4kN/m (Kerdok *et al.*, 2002). As mentioned previously, the authors found that running mechanics remained unchanged due to increases in leg stiffness as surface stiffness decreased. Rebound height during drop jumps has also been shown to increase on softer surfaces (Arampatzis *et al.*, 2004) despite greater absolute energy loss. This further emphasises the importance of incorporating the entire athlete–surface system when considering the influence of energy storage and return on performance.

Unfortunately the exact physiological mechanism that is responsible for increased performance when the overall system stiffness (combined surface and leg stiffness) is optimised is unknown but different possible factors have been proposed. Changes to the timing and magnitude of the stretch shortening cycle could allow for greater internal energy storage in structures like the Achilles tendon (Bosco *et al.*, 1997), which has been proposed to have a large influence on performance (Alexander and Bennett, 1989). An improved mechanical advantage (Ferris and Farley, 1997) due to reduced leg flexion has also been proposed. The straighter leg would require lower muscle forces (Biewener, 1989) and the possibility of muscles working more isometrically with decreased shortening distances and velocities resulting in reduced muscle work (Kerdok *et al.*, 2002). Further research is required to determine exactly how surface stiffness interacts with the athlete to optimise the musculoskeletal system and maximise performance.

## Key summary points

- Traction can have a large influence on performance.
- Increases in performance only occur until a certain critical threshold that is dictated by the athlete's utilised traction.
- Further increases in available traction above this threshold will not influence performance since athletes cannot utilise any more of the available traction.
- Alterations of surfaces can influence traction, however a lack of in-depth studies have failed to show whether these alterations in surface characteristics and traction are large enough to alter performance.
- Energy storage and return in sports surfaces can influence athletic performance.
- To improve performance, energy should be returned at the proper location, in the right direction, at the correct time with the appropriate frequency.

- Sports surface compliance can influence performance by modifying how an athlete's muscles generate force.

## References


Alexander, R. M. and Bennett, M. B. (1989) 'How elastic is a running shoe?', *New Scientist*, 123: 45–46.

Arampatzis, A., Bruggemann, G. and Metzler, V. (1999) 'The effect of speed on leg stiffness depends on knee stiffness during human running', *Journal of Biomechanics,* 32: 1349–1353.

Arampatzis, A., Bruggemann, G. and Klapsing, G. (2001) 'Leg stiffness and mechanical energetic processes during jumping on a sprung surface', *Medicine and Science in Sports and Exercise*, 33: 923–931.

Arampatzis, A., Stafilidis, S., Morey-Klapsing, G. and Bruggemann, G.-P. (2004) 'Interaction of the human body and surfaces of different stiffness during drop jumps', *Medicine and Science in Sports and Exercise*, 36: 451–459.

Baroud, G., Nigg, B. M. and Stefanyshyn, D. J. (1999a) 'Energy storage and return in sport surfaces', *Sports Engineering*, 2: 173–180.

Baroud, G., Nigg, B. M. and Stefanyshyn, D. J. (1999b) 'Can athletic performance be enhanced by sport surfaces and sport shoes?', *Proceedings of the International Society of Biomechanics XVIIth Congress*, 237.

Biewener, A. A. (1989) 'Scaling body support in mammals: Limb posture and muscle mechanics', *Science*, 245: 45–48.

Bonstingl, R. W., Morehouse, C. A. and Niebel, B. W. (1975) 'Torques developed by different types of shoes on various playing surfaces', *Medicine and Science in Sports and Exercise*, 7: 127–131.

Bosco, C., Saggini, R. and Viru, A. (1997) 'The influence of different floor stiffness on mechanical efficiency of leg extensor muscle', *Ergonomics*, 40: 670–679.

Farley, C. T., Houdijk, H. H., Van Strien, C. and Louie, M. (1998) 'Mechanism of leg stiffness adjustment for hopping on surfaces of different stiffnesses', *Journal of Applied Physiology*, 85: 1044–1055.

Ferris, D. P. and Farley, C. T. (1997) 'Interaction of leg stiffness and surfaces stiffness during human hopping', *Journal of Applied Physiology,* 82: 15–22.

Ferris, D. P., Louie, M. and Farley, C. T. (1998) 'Running in the real world: adjusting leg stiffness for different surfaces', *Proceedings of the Royal Society of London: Biological Sciences*, 265: 989–994.

Ferris, D. P., Liang, K. and Farley, C. T. (1999) 'Runners adjust leg stiffness for their first step on a new running surface', *Journal of Biomechanics*, 32: 787–794.

Fleming, P. (2011) 'Artificial turf systems for sport surfaces: Current knowledge and research needs', *Proceedings of the Institution of Mechanical Engineers, Part P: Journal of Sports Engineering and Technology*, 225(2): 43–63.

Ford, K., Manson, N., Evans, B., Myer, G., Gwin, R., Heidt, R. and Hewett, T. (2006) 'Comparison of in-shoe foot loading patterns on natural grass and synthetic turf', *Journal of Science and Medicine in Sport*, 9(6): 433–40.

Gains, G. L., Swedenhjelm, A. N., Mayhew, J. L., Bird, H. M. and Houser, J. J. (2010) 'Comparison of speed and agility performance of college football players on field turf and natural grass', *Journal of Strength and Conditioning Research*, 24(10): 2613.

Hardin, E. C., van den Bogert, A. J. and Hamill, J. (2004) 'Kinematic adaptations during running: Effects of footwear, surface, and duration', *Medicine and Science in Sports and Exercise*, 36: 838–844.

Ker, R. F., Bennett, M. B., Bibby, S. R., Kester, R. C. and Alexander, R. M. (1987) 'The spring in the arch of the human foot', *Nature*, 325: 147–149.

Kerdok, A. E., Biewener, A. A., McMahon, T. A., Weyand, P. G. and Herr, H. M. (2002) 'Energetics and mechanics of human running on surfaces of different stiffnesses', *Journal of Applied Physiology*, 92: 469–478.

Lambson, R., Barnhill, B. and Higgins, R. (1996) 'Football cleat design and its effect on anterior cruciate ligament injuries: A three year prospective study', *American Journal of Sports Medicine*, 24(2): 155–159.

Livesay, G., Reda, D. and Nauman, E. (2006) 'Peak torque and rotational stiffness developed at the shoe–surface interface: The effect of shoe and playing surface', *American Journal of Sports Medicine*, 34: 415–422.

Luo, G. and Stefanyshyn, D. (2011) 'Identification of critical traction values for maximum athletic performance', *Footwear Science*, 3(3): 127–138.

McMahon, T. A. and Greene, P. R. (1978) 'Fast running tracks', *Scientific American*, 239: 112–121.

McMahon, T. A. and Greene, P. R. (1979) 'The influence of track compliance on running', *Journal of Biomechanics*, 12: 893–904.

Moritz, C. T. and Farley, C. T. (2005) 'Human hopping on very soft elastic surfaces: Implications for muscle pre-stretch and elastic energy storage in locomotion', *Journal of Experimental Biology*, 208: 939–949.

Nigg, B. M. (1999) 'Force', *Biomechanics of the Musculoskeletal System*. New York, NY: John Wiley and Sons, pp. 261–287.

Nigg, B. M. and Anton, M. (1995) 'Energy aspects for elastic and viscous shoe soles and playing surfaces', *Medicine and Science in Sports and Exercise*, 27: 92–97.

Nigg, B. M. and Segesser, B. (1992) 'Biomechanical and orthopedic concepts in sport shoe construction', *Medicine and Science in Sports and Exercise*, 24: 595–602.

Nigg, B. M. and Yeadon, M. R. (1987) 'Biomechanical aspects of playing surfaces', *Journal of Sports Sciences*, 5: 117–145.

Potthast, W. (2010) 'Motion differences in goal kicking on natural and artificial soccer turf systems', *Footwear Science*, 2(1): 29–35.

Potthast, W., Verhelst, R., Hughes, M., Stone, K. and De Clercq, D. (2010) 'Football-specific evaluation of player–surface interaction on different football turf systems', *Sports Technology*, 3(1): 5–12.

Sanders, R. H. and Allen, J. B. (1993) 'Changes in net joint torques during accommodation to change in surface compliance in a drop jumping task', *Human Movement Sciences*, 12: 299–326.

Severn, K. A., Fleming, P. R. and Dixon, N. (2010) 'Science of synthetic turf surfaces: player–surface interactions', *Sports Technology*, 3(1): 13–25.

Severn, K. A., Fleming, P. R., Clarke, J. D. and Carre, M. J. (2011) 'Science of synthetic turf surfaces: Investigating traction behavior', *Proceedings of the Institution of Mechanical Engineers, Part P: Journal of Sports Engineering and Technology*, 225(3): 147–158.

Stafilidis, S. and Arampatzis, A. (2007) 'Track compliance does not affect sprinting performance', *Journal of Sports Sciences*, 25(13): 1479–1490.

Stanitski, C., McMaster, J. and Ferguson, R. (1974) 'Synthetic turf and grass: A comparative study', *The American Journal of Sports Medicine*, 2(1): 22–26.

Stefanyshyn, D. J. and Nigg, B. M. (2000) *International Handbook of Sport Science, Biomechanics and Biology of Human Movement*. Champaign, IL: Human Kinetics Publishers, pp. 49–66.

Sterzing, T., Hennig, E. and Milani, T. (2007) 'Biomechanical requirements of soccer shoe construction', *Orthopadie Technik*, 58(9): 646–655.

Torg, J., Quedenfeld, T. and Landau, S. (1974) 'The shoe–surface interface and its relationship to football knee injuries', *The American Journal of Sports Medicine*, 2(5): 261–269.

Verhelst, R. (2010) *Study of Ball–Surface and Player–Surface Interaction on Artificial Turf*, Doctoral dissertation, Ghent University, Belgium.

Villwock, M. R., Meyer, E. G., Powell, J. W., Fouty, A. J. and Haut, R. C. (2009a) 'Football playing surface and shoe design affect rotational traction', *The American Journal of Sports Medicine*, 37(3): 518–525.

Villwock, M. R., Meyer, E. G., Powell, J. W., Fouty, A. J. and Haut, R. C. (2009b) 'The effects of various infills, fibre structures, and shoe designs on generating rotational traction on an artificial surface', *Proceedings of the Institution of Mechanical Engineers, Part P: Journal of Sports Engineering and Technology*, 223: 11–19.

Wannop, J. W. and Stefanyshyn, D. J. (2012) 'The effect of normal load, speed and moisture on footwear traction', *Footwear Science*, 4(1): 37–43.

Worobets, J. T. and Wannop, J. W. (2012) 'Influence of shoe mass, traction and forefoot stiffness on athletic performance', *Medicine and Science in Sports and Exercise*, submitted (ID MSSE-D-12-00210).

Young, C. (2006) *Performance of Water-based Hockey Pitches*, Doctoral dissertation, Loughborough University, UK.

Chapter 6

# Mechanical aspects of shoe–surface interaction

*Matt Carré, James Clarke and Paul Fleming*

## Introduction

When considering shoe–surface interactions the 'traction' developed can be defined as the horizontal force that resists movement between the contacting components while the shoe is loaded (note: the interaction between a non-studded shoe and surfaces is also referred to simply as 'friction'). Traction can be generated through a number of differing tribological and mechanical interactions, including combinations, largely dependent on two broad categories of footwear, studded and non-studded. The loading normal to the surface, and the consequent 'force reduction' during a movement is also a key factor and the methods to test this have been discussed in Chapter 3. Severn *et al.* (2011) highlight the requirement for improved scientific understanding of the different interactions at the sports shoe–surface interface and this will aid in the improved design of playing surfaces and footwear constructions.

During dynamic sport-specific movements such as accelerating, braking, turning and side-stepping the traction developed at the shoe–surface interface is critical to injury risk and performance of the player (Frederick, 1986). As outlined in Chapter 4, too much or too little traction can lead to injury and there is often a suggested acceptable range (Milburn and Barry, 1998). Excessive traction may result in an injury caused by overloading in the lower extremities. Insufficient traction will cause a slip, or even a fall which may cause injury itself. Many studies have identified risk factors in sport and view shoe–surface traction as an extrinsic injury risk factor (Powell and Shootman, 1992; Murphy *et al.*, 2003; Andersen *et al.*, 2003; Arnason *et al.*, 2004; Griffin *et al.*, 2006). Following an epidemiological study into the incidence of soccer injury, Volpi (2008) stated surface and footwear as primary injury risk factors for soccer players. Excessive rotational resistance at the shoe–surface interface has been identified as an injury risk factor, therefore sufficiently low traction is desired to reduce the stresses experienced in an athlete's lower extremities (Durá, 1999) (see Chapters 4 and 7 for more detail on biomechanics, injury and human–surface interactions).

As described in Chapter 5, traction also affects performance, as athletes require sufficient traction to accelerate and decelerate rapidly. An optimum shoe–surface combination will therefore often provide a balance of sufficiently high translational traction (performance), and sufficiently low rotational traction (player safety). Understanding the interactions between footwear and surfaces will help players choose the optimum footwear to balance performance with injury risk. There is therefore a requirement to understand how the shoe and the surface interact, in order to provide an optimum balance of performance and injury risk in sport.

This chapter examines the mechanical aspects of shoe–surface interactions, firstly discussing how key player movements have been simulated by researchers and then considering in detail the two categories of studded and non-studded footwear–surface interactions.

## Simulation of key movements

Frederick (1986) highlighted the need to develop repeatable test methods to quantify the range of traction that will allow high performance and acceptable injury risk in sport and a number of mechanical methods have been developed over recent years. Most attempt to simulate a sports-specific biomechanical movement and involve the rotation or translation of a loaded test shoe, or a combination of both, relative to a surface. Mechanical test devices have the advantage of creating objective loading conditions that provide a repeatable measure of shoe–surface traction, eliminating the inherent uncertainties that exist when subject testing is employed.

Improved biomechanical measurement techniques and necessary actuator and transducer technology have led to sophisticated mechanical test devices that replicate the specific loading conditions that athletes experience during play, to a large extent. For example, Grund *et al.* (2007) and Grund and Senner (2010) analysed TV sequences of soccer players leading up to real ACL injuries. The resulting kinematic data was used to develop a multi-body computer simulation with a simplified human body model to determine an approximation of the loads that occur during a real injury situation. This information was evaluated in order to develop a prototype mechanical test rig which replicates the full range of motion during a real injury situation. A pneumatic control unit applies a force to push an artificial leg into the surface, and, at the same time, an appropriate rotational force is applied along the longitudinal axis of the leg. The internal transmittable loads are measured by a six-component load cell.

### *Extracting relevant measures of traction*

Once the shoe–surface interaction is understood from a biomechanical perspective and a suitable test device has been developed, the relevant measures can be extracted from the resulting force data. Different movements require the understanding of different traction mechanisms, e.g. straight-line sprinting in soccer may require the study of the 'give' in the surface when pushing off, while gross sliding on clay tennis courts would require measures of dynamic traction. The changing relationships between traction force, displacement and time, during a traction test, depend entirely on the shoe, surface and loading used, but Table 6.1 summarises some common measurements of translation traction used in shoe–surface interaction research.

An example of a typical trace of force against displacement from a recent study on tennis is shown in Figure 6.1. This particular plot is characterised by two particular regions: a) a region of increasing initial force during a static regime, ending with a coinciding static and peak traction force; b) a period of dynamic traction during which the force remains relatively constant.

*Table 6.1* A summary of different measurements of translational traction commonly used.

| | *Definition* | *Explanation* | *One example showing relevance* |
|---|---|---|---|
| Traction force | Static traction force | The force required to initiate *significant* movement of the shoe. | The point at which a soccer player would lose their footing in a push-off. |
| | Peak traction force | The peak force measured during an entire movement. Sometimes this is the same as the static traction force. | The maximum reaction force provided during scrimmaging for a rugby player. |
| | Dynamic traction force | The mean force required for the shoe to keep moving through the surface over a period of time/displacement. | The general force opposing motion and slowing down a tennis player during a slide on clay. |
| | Initial 'stiffness' | The force required for the shoe to move a pre-determined displacement, divided by that displacement. | The 'response' experienced by a sprinter leading to improved performance. |

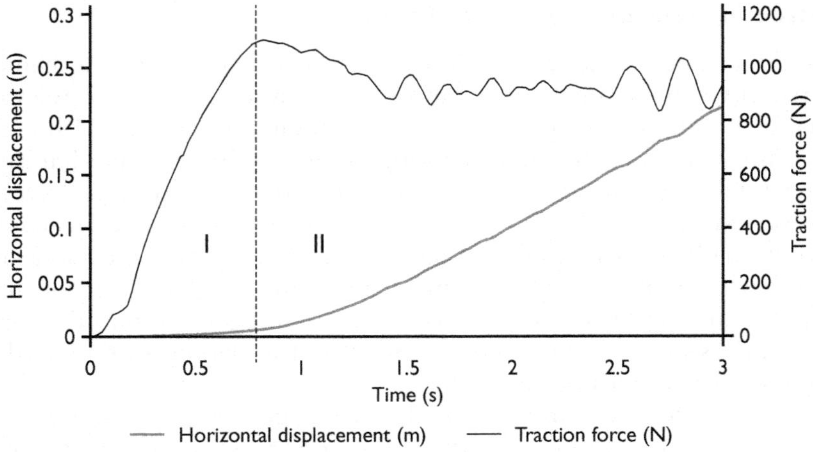


*Figure 6.1* A typical plot of traction force and displacement against time when driving a loaded test shoe across a wet artificial clay tennis surface, reproduced with kind permission from Clarke *et al.* (2013a).

## Studded footwear–surface interactions

This section is concerned with the various mechanical interactions that relate to translational and rotational traction between studded footwear and sports surfaces. In various versions of 'football', including association (soccer), American, rugby and Australian rules, studded footwear (sometimes referred to as 'cleated') is worn by players to aid the traction they receive from the playing surface during a movement. Other sports, such as athletics, golf and cricket all use different forms of spiked footwear, which may lead to similar traction mechanisms, but these will not be discussed in detail here. The interaction between studded footwear and sports surfaces is a complex system and cannot be described by Coloumb's classical laws of friction (Shorten *et al.*, 2003). Depending on the situation the resistance to movement of a studded shoe through a turf system can be made up of: the effects of surface friction between shoe materials (e.g. the sole plate and studs) and the parts of the turf system with which they are in contact (e.g. fibres, grass, rubber in-fill, roots, soil etc.); 'ploughing' forces due to the necessary movement of in-fill particles; plastic deformation of soil; and changes in the stud–surface interaction during the movement, such as depth of penetration.

These traction mechanisms and the consequent overall traction force will therefore be dependent on the characteristics of the footwear, and also the surface make-up and conditions.

### *Artificial surfaces*

The development and introduction of third-generation artificial turfs surfaces with an in-fill of sand and rubber particles, stimulated much research into studded footwear–surface interactions. In comparison with first- and second-generation surfaces, third-generation artificial turfs have longer fibres which are more spread out, and are manufactured from polymers (such as polypropylene or polyethylene) found to be less abrasive to the skin. Developments in manufacturing processes have led to various fibre designs including monofilament fibres which are individually produced and twisted together, and fibrillated fibres which have a honeycomb structure in order to prevent infill migration (see Chapter 2 for more details).

### *Natural surfaces*

Natural sport surfaces are complex surface systems comprising of granular soil material (made up of sand, silt and clay particles) and a grass plant (Guisasola *et al.*, 2009). The tractional behaviour of a natural turf system has been found to be affected by a number of surface system and environmental variables – these are: particle make-up (termed 'mineralogy'); ground cover; grass species; grass root length and density; grass length; compaction; bulk density; temperature; and moisture content (Baker, 1990, 1991; Canaway and Baker, 1993; Canaway *et al.*, 1990; Orchard, 2001, 2001; Orchard *et al.*, 1999; Guisasola *et al.* 2009). Although advances in understanding the behaviour of natural turf systems have been made, the high number of variables makes understanding the effects of an individual variable on player traction difficult. Orchard (2001) hypothesised a relationship model between surface traction, surface hardness, ground conditions and stud length (Figure 6.2). A common link between the aforementioned studies is the controlling effect moisture content has on soil strength and failure mechanisms. More information relating to natural surfaces is provided in Chapter 8.

### *Research into studded footwear mechanisms*

Examining the traction of studded footwear requires an understanding of the combination of effects associated with the shoe, the surface, the loading conditions and the mechanical traction test rig employed. There are challenges in directly comparing results from different studies as the mechanical test methods vary greatly in design, in particular the loading conditions and the driving mechanism. This is highlighted in Table 6.2, which summarises a number of methods used in recent studies investigating studded footwear. However, general key findings and considerations for future work can be extracted.

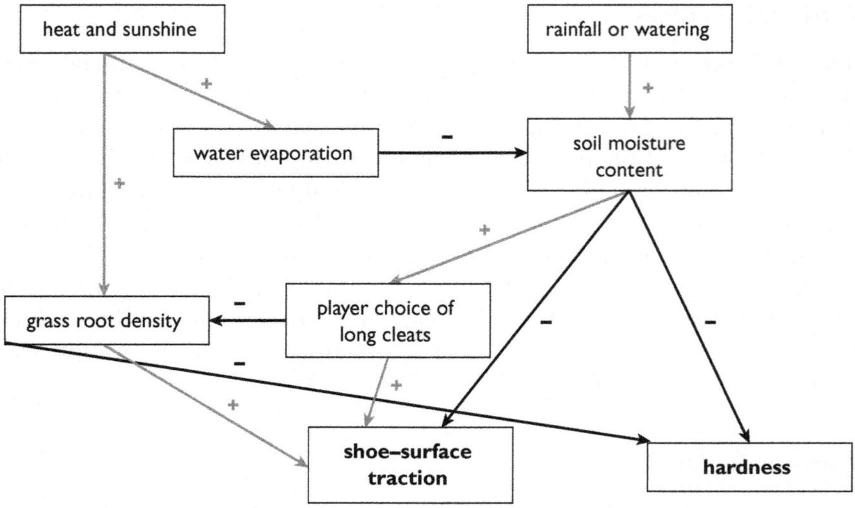


*Figure 6.2* Relationship between hardness, boot–surface traction and ground conditions, reproduced with kind permission from Orchard (2001). In this study studs were termed 'cleats'.

Shorten *et al.* (2003) used the mechanical testing method described in Table 6.2 to compare the traction of 24 shoe–surface combinations. The four surfaces in the study were a dry natural turf, a conventional second-generation synthetic turf with 10mm pile height and sand infill, and two third-generation synthetic turfs with pile heights of 50mm. One had a 40mm infill of rubber, and the other had a 40mm infill of rubber and sand. The outsole of the six shoes tested varied from a typical basketball shoe with no studs to a heavily studded American football shoe. The translational and rotational traction were both measured using an Exeter Research Shoe and Surface Traction Tester (Exeter Research Inc., Exeter, NH, USA). The translational traction was characterised as the coefficient of traction (COT), the ratio of horizontal force and vertical force, at the 'initial period' of movement. The rotational traction was characterised as the peak moment resisting rotation. The results highlighted how trends can vary between surfaces. The second-generation turf had the lowest mean translational traction but the highest resistance to rotation, making shoe selection on this surface difficult. Both third-generation surfaces had higher translational traction values than the natural turf but lower rotational resistance. The third-generation artificial surface with exclusively rubber infill gave the highest mean translational traction, but lowest rotational traction, highlighting infill material will affect traction.

Vachon (2004) compared three typical stud types: dimpled studs, moulded studs and bladed studs, on three surfaces (a natural surface, a five year-old third-generation turf with infill and a third-generation turf without infill). On the natural surface it was found that the rotational traction and translational traction, measured as the mean peak torque and peak coefficient of traction respectively, were independent of sole type. The infilled surface exhibited the highest mean peak torque for the moulded sole, but there was no statistically significant difference between the moulded and bladed soles. There was, however, a significant difference between the moulded and pimpled soles, with moulded soles giving higher torque. The surface without an infill, showed significant reductions in mean rotational resistance, compared to that with the infill for both the bladed and moulded soles (from 33 to 24Nm and 36 to 28Nm, respectively). There was, however, a significant increase for the pimple design, from 29 to 36Nm. The translational traction showed no difference between sole type for the infilled artificial surface and natural turf. Without an infill, the pimple design experienced a higher coefficient of traction (1.1) than both the moulded (0.81) and bladed designs (0.7).

The differences found between the infill and non-infill surfaces highlight the unpredictable interaction between surface and studded shoe. Interestingly the longer studded shoes (moulds and blades) saw a significant increase in both translational traction and rotational resistance on artificial turf with an infill; however a pimple design gave the highest values on the surface without an infill. The extra traction force experienced may be a result of the higher penetration depth of the moulded and bladed studs into the infilled surface. This highlights the need to measure stud penetration/vertical displacement and quantify its effect on traction.

Vachon (2004) states that the fibre density and material must affect the adhesion, and therefore the traction, provided by artificial surfaces. The softer, rubber pimple stud offers more surface friction via adhesion to the synthetic fibres of artificial surfaces, when compared to studs made of harder materials, and therefore provides greater traction. This influence of adhesion may have contributed to the unpredictable behaviour of the two artificial surfaces tested. Livesay *et al.* (2006) used similar apparatus to Vachon (2004) to measure the rotational traction of the forefoot of two separate loaded shoes – a 'grass' shoe with 10 studs on the forefoot, of length 12.7mm, and a 'turf' shoe with a dimpled pattern, maximum height in profile of 9.5mm. They examined a natural turf, three separate third-generation artificial turfs of same pile length but different infill material, and also a second-generation AstroTurf surface with both shoe types. A comparison of their results is shown in Figure 6.3.

Livesay *et al.* (2006) reported differences in peak torques and rotational traction between artificial surfaces with differing infill make-up. For both shoe types tested ('grass' and 'turf'), the artificial surface with exclusively rubber infill experienced the highest mean peak torque (between 0 and 2 degrees rotation), in comparison to a 50 per cent sand and 50 per cent

*Table 6.2* A summary of methods and findings from recent studies (starting with most recent).

| *Study* | *Test device* | *Driving force* | *Loading method* | *Loading condition* | *Measure extracted* | *Key findings* | *Suggested future work* |
|---|---|---|---|---|---|---|---|
| Severn *et al.* (2011) | Translational | Device 1: Pneumatic ram, increasing force | Hydraulic ram | 250 to 450N | Traction force over 50mm travel | Traction force is greatly influenced by changes in the normal force for all test methods used and also the spacing of studs (relative to the pivot point) for peak rotational traction (from Device 2). | Future studies need to incorporate more information on the surface material behaviour and state. The development of mechanical test apparatus are is required that better simulates human loading (magnitude and rates) and provide continuous measurement of load, displacement, and vertical penetration/compression during testing. |
| | | Device 2: Pneumatic ram, controlled Velocity (10mm/s) | Weights | 440 to 640N | Traction force over 50mm travel | | |
| | Rotational | Rotated by hand | Weights | 450N | Peak torque | Device 2 showed an increase in both the peak rotational and peak translational traction resistance for an increase in the bulk density of the rubber infill. | |
| | | Device 2: Pneumatic ram, controlled rotational velocity (12 deg°/s) | Weights | 440 to 640N | Torque, up to 60 deg° | Stud penetration (using Device 1) was found to be influenced by vertical load and the rubber infill thickness. | |
| Villwock *et al.* (2010) | Dynamic Rotation | Weighted (425N) pendulum at 180 deg/s) | Weights | 1000N vertical (95th percentile male during a sports activity) | Peak Torque<br>Rotational Stiffness | Most shoe-surface interface values in the current study exceeded this threshold level set in the 1970s. | The effects of moisture and temperature on traction characteristics of infill-based artificial surfaces need additional study. |

| *Study* | *Test device* | *Driving force* | *Loading method* | *Loading condition* | *Measure extracted* | *Key findings* | *Suggested future work* |
|---|---|---|---|---|---|---|---|
| Grund *et al.* (2010) | Rotational | Pneumatic 'muscle' (45Nm to 130Nm) | Pneumatic | 1000N–2450N axial loading | Peak Torque and Effective (dynamic) Torque | Heavily studded shoes did not produce higher torques. The nature of the loading significantly influences the result. | Analysis of data from further loading scenarios is required. |
| Rosa *et al.* (2007) | Translational (Horizontal displacement) | Controlled Velocity (0.4m/s) | Pneumatic | 150N vertical | Peak COT | Maintenance operations influence traction on natural surfaces. | A subjective study is required to relate traction requirements. |
| Livesay *et al.* (2006) | Rotational | Rotated by hand (minimum 75 deg) | Weights | 67, 111, 200, 333, and 511N. Results were analysed at the 333N condition | Peak torque, rotation stiffness (Nm/deg) after 2 deg and 10 deg) | Low peak torques found on the natural surface in comparison with artificial. Studs changed trends in initial stiffness found between the traction experienced on surfaces. | Further understanding of the traction measured by mechanical methods is required. |
| Vachon (2004) | Rotational | Rotated by hand | Weights | 441N | Peak torque required to initiate movement | A surface without infill can offer the same torque as a natural surface while obtaining an equivalent or superior friction coefficient. | Traction testing requires using a broad range of outsoles when assessing a surface. |
| | Translational | Pulled by hand | Weights | 156N | Peak force | | |
| Shorten *et al.* (2003) | Translational | Variable speed electric motor (max speed = 0.3m/s) | Weights | 529N | Average ratio of horizontal and vertical force during initial period | Surfaces with granular infills (3G) showed higher translational and lower rotational traction than the 2G surface tested. | Further understanding of how the make-up of 3G artificial surfaces affects traction is required. |
| | Rotational | Pulled by hand | Weights | 529N | Peak force | | |

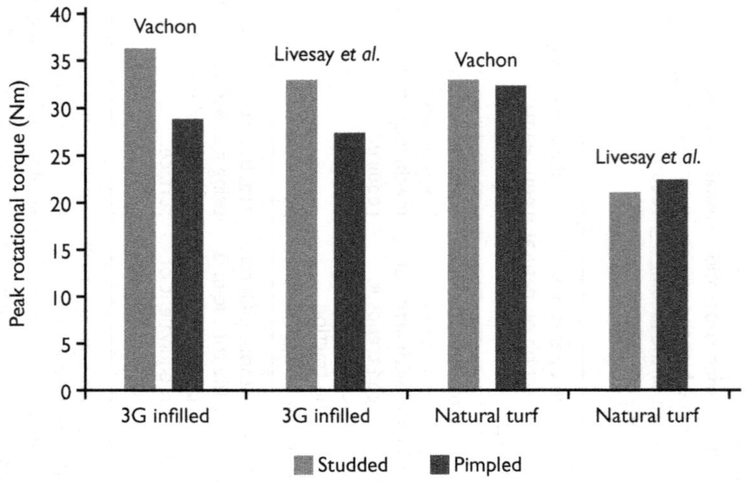


*Figure 6.3* A comparison of mean rotational torques from the studies by Vachon (2004) and Livesay *et al.* (2006).

rubber infill and a 70 per cent rubber and 30 per cent sand infill. The torque was sampled throughout rotation and it was found that the 100 per cent rubber infilled surface experienced the lowest mean rotational traction force later in the rotation (between 2 and 10 degrees). For this range of traction the force increased as the sand content increased. This highlights the importance of replicating the conditions of real human movements in order to determine a reliable and realistic comparable measure.

When considering mean peak rotational torque the three third-generation artificial turfs produced significantly higher values than the natural surface with the studded 'grass' shoe, suggesting an increased risk in ACL injury. Consistent with previous studies discussed, the 'grass' shoe, which has longer but fewer studs, gave higher peak torque values, than the more pimpled 'turf' shoe, particularly on the artificial turfs. This indicates that both the shoe and the surface type contribute to injury risk and may explain why Meyers and Barnhill (2004) found (over a five-year study) a greater number of ACL trauma injuries on natural turf when compared to a third-generation sand and rubber-infilled artificial turf (presuming shoe choice was affected by surface type).

Shorten *et al.* (2003) argue against using heavily studded shoes during play as the higher rotational resistance they are likely to give is associated with an increase in noncontact ACL injuries. Valiant (1990) argues that the rotational traction available should be reduced to a minimum, as rotational traction does not offer any athletic advantage. Lambson *et al.* (1996) conducted a three-year study comparing the rotational resistance of four shoe types with recorded injury data from players wearing the same shoes. The results show a significant increase of ACL injuries with players wearing shoes with an 'edge' stud design, that have large studs around the edge of the shoe and smaller studs elsewhere. When mechanically tested, these shoes also had significantly higher rotational resistance when compared to three other stud designs. These findings correspond with González *et al.* (2003), who found that studs on the edge of soccer boots experience higher forces during running and cutting movements when compared to studs nearer the centre of the forefront. Arguably, smaller studs on the edge of the shoe and larger studs in the centre of the shoe could optimise the traction given from a studded shoe by reducing rotational resistance while maintaining translational traction.

The variations in forces between different shoe–surface combinations demonstrate the need to select appropriate footwear for the given surface condition and the difficulties in predicting shoe–surface interaction. The results found by Vachon (2004) and Shorten *et al.* (2003) strengthen the argument for testing translational and rotational traction for a studded shoe–surface combination independently. Figure 6.4 shows neither study found a relationship between rotational and translational traction. This may be due to the different methodologies used in determining translational and rotational traction. Vachon (2004) measured peak horizontal force and peak torque to measure translational and rotational traction respectively. As peak readings were taken for both measures of traction a linear relationship might be expected. However, the normal load applied to the footwear during each test differed. A force of 441N was applied during translational testing and a force of 156N was applied during rotational traction testing. The differences in normal loading will influence the traction mechanisms developed at the boot–surface interface. As normal load increases the stud penetration is likely to increase, therefore changes to the friction forces from the outsole-surface contact and the ploughing traction associated with the studs displacing the surface material will have clouded any potential relationships between rotational and translational traction. Shorten *et al.* (2003) used very different mechanical devices to measure translational and rotational traction in their study. Translational traction was measured as the initial mean dynamic force as a motor pulled the footwear across a surface at a speed of 0.3m/s. Rotational traction was measured as the peak torque, via a torque wrench being rotated by hand. Although the normal force applied was the same for each test (529N) the differences between the testing methodologies conducted, and the measures of traction extracted, may explain why no relationship between translational and rotational traction was found (see Figure 6.4).

The results from both of these studies show the difficulties in predicting surface characteristics and behaviour. Ideally, each shoe–surface

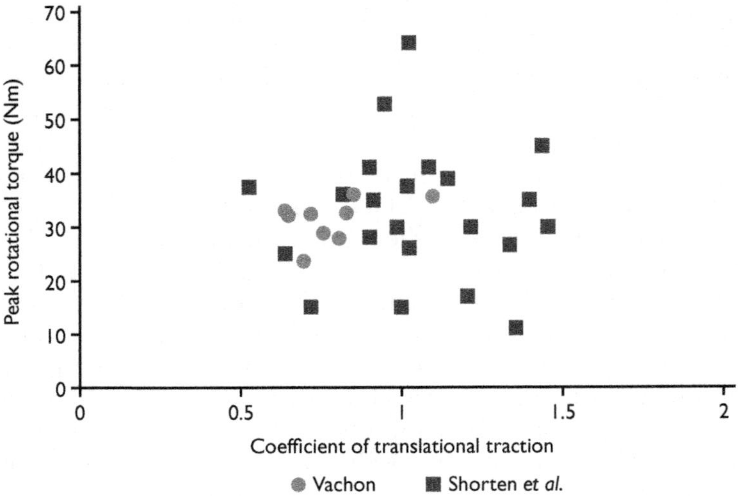


*Figure 6.4* Mean translational and rotational traction for individual shoe and surface combinations from Vachon (2004) and Shorten *et al.* (2003).

combination needs to be examined individually to understand its particular interaction.

The force applied to the studded outsole contrasts between studies. Rosa *et al.* (2007) applied a normal force of 150N for mechanical translational traction tests. When comparing friction-measuring methods, Wojcieszak *et al.* (1997) applied a vertical load of 696N when using an Exeter Research Shoe and Surface Traction Tester with basketball shoes. Shorten *et al.* (2003), however, applied 529N when using the same traction tester to compare studded footwear. When testing the traction of studded golf shoes, Williams and Neugebauer (2007) applied 250N to the forefront of each test shoe. Vachon (2004) applied 159N for translational traction tests and 441N during rotational traction tests. Severn *et al.* (2011) used a range of normal loads in the four test methods but included a benchmarking value of approximately 450N. When testing rotational traction, Livesay *et al.* (2006) found a significant linear relationship between the vertical force applied to the test shoe (67, 111, 200, 333, and 511N) and initial stiffness and peak torque. The test device was limited to 511N; therefore they decided to use a midrange 333N vertical force. Severn *et al.* (2011) also found a linear trend between peak rotational traction force and normal load.

The studies reviewed show the factors involved and the difficulties mechanical tests have in predicting shoe–surface traction. For mechanical test devices to realistically predict surface–shoe interaction there is a need for further development of current techniques and to incorporate an understanding of surface properties. Mechanical test devices must attempt to replicate the forces and velocities that appear in player movements (see Chapter 7). Any test device which does not accurately represent an actual loading condition cannot predict the effects of shoe and surface parameters on the injury risk or performance of an athlete.

When mechanically testing shoe–surface traction particular consideration must also be given to understanding the characteristics and condition of the surface during testing. Table 6.3 highlights the large number of key independent variables associated with mechanical traction testing of studded soccer boots on natural and artificial playing surfaces identified from the extant literature. By identifying the associated parameters of shoe–surface interaction it is possible to understand the traction mechanisms at stud–surface contact. The studies reviewed here often compared the traction of artificial surfaces to a natural surface; however, the characteristics of each surface are often ill-defined. There is, in general, a lack of quantified published research data for surface properties and traction, particularly for artificial third-generation turf surfaces (Severn *et al.*, 2011).

As highlighted in Table 6.3 traction is dependent on a number of stud parameters. Stud penetration, defined as the vertical displacement of the stud(s), will have a significant effect on the traction measured and is dependent on the geometric parameters associated with the studded outsole, but is also affected by the surface's compressive strength and shear strength. Therefore the resistance to stud penetration of a natural soccer surface is dependent on a number of factors associated with the soil make-up: density; moisture content; and particle make-up. Similarly, an artificial surface's resistance to stud penetration will be dependent on the factors associated with its infill, fibre density and tufts.

Clarke (2011) found that natural turf that had low moisture content resulted in low penetration and hence low traction, whereas high moisture content resulted in high penetration, but still low traction as excessive moisture in the turf can then act as a lubricant. High traction was only measured on the turf samples with moisture content in between the two extremes.

Clarke (2011) also carried out a parametric traction study on four different third-generation artificial turfs using 13 bespoke stud geometries that varied in length, average diameter and conicity. The traction force measured did not significantly differ when larger studs were used. This was found to be due to the level of penetration obtained (i.e. larger studs can provide greater ploughing traction, but only if they can be penetrated fully into the surface). Penetration was found to correlate with the stud geometry parameters (length, width and conicity) but the surface make-up also affected the mechanism of the traction observed. For instance, the ploughing traction in surfaces with lower density infill was lower, and

*Table 6.3* A summary of key variables associated with mechanical traction testing of studded soccer boots.

| | | | | | |
|---|---|---|---|---|---|
| Playing surface | Third-generation artificial soccer surface | Fibre | Material | Polypropylene | |
| | | | | Polyethylene | |
| | | | Type | Monofilament | |
| | | | | Fibrillated | |
| | | | Dimensions | Width | |
| | | | | Thickness | |
| | | | | Length | |
| | | Tufts | Total number | | |
| | | | Number of fibres per tuft | | |
| | | | Density (tufts/area) | | |
| | | Infill | Type | Rubber crumb | Density (mass/area) |
| | | | | Sand | Ratio of each |
| | | | Depth | | |
| | | | Particle size | | |
| | | | Particle shape | | |
| | Natural soccer surface | Soil moisture content | | | |
| | | Bulk density (g/m3) | | | |
| | | Particle make up of soil | % of clay, sand and silt content. | | |
| | | Grass species | | | |
| | | Organic matter | Root density | | |
| | | | Grass cover | | |
| | | | Grass length | | |
| | | Environmental characteristics | Temperature | | |
| | | | Water evaporation rates | | |
| | | | Water infiltration rates | | |
| | | | Foreign contaminants | | |

| | | | | |
|---|---|---|---|---|
| Studded outsole | Studs | Geometry | Length | |
| | | | Width | |
| | | | Conical | |
| | | | Volume | |
| | | | Cross sectional area | |
| | | Configuration | Number of studs | |
| | | | Spacing between studs | |
| | | Material properties | Coefficient of friction | |
| | Outsole | Material properties | Coefficient of friction | |
| | | | Stiffness | |
| | | Contact area | | |
| | | Orientation to the surface | Linear | |
| | | | Lateral | |
| | | | Angled | |
| Mechanics of traction testing device | Loading conditions | | Force applied (N) | |
| | | | Orientation of the force | Normal to the surface |
| | | | | Oblique to the surface |
| | Loading method | | Pneumatic | |
| | | | Hydraulic | |
| | | | Weights | |
| | | | Gravity (e.g. pendulum/ramp) | |
| | Driving mechanism | | Force-controlled | Pneumatic |
| | | | | Hydraulic |
| | | | | Pulled by hand |
| | | | Velocity-controlled | Motorised (constant velocity) |

therefore the traction significantly reduced when the studs were not fully penetrated and contact was lost between the outsole plate and the surface, further reducing the frictional resistance to movement. This effect was not found with a surface with high density of infill, where the ploughing traction was the dominant component of traction.

These final studies illustrate the sometimes complex interaction of all the variables involved but show that for studded shoes to perform correctly, it is vital that the studs are able to penetrate fully into the surface. This minimum requirement drives the alternative standard designs available, such as a 'soft ground' boot with a small number of relatively long studs and a 'hard ground' boot with a larger number of relatively short studs.

## Non-studded footwear-surface interactions

On non-studded footwear, a rubber compound, or a similarly viscoelastic material, is generally used on the outsoles, often with some kind of 'tread' or pattern. In clean, dry conditions, sliding contacts between viscoelastic materials and a hard solid substrate will result in a combination of adhesive and hysteretic friction mechanisms and also abrasive wear (Gronqvist *et al.*, 2003; Persson, 2001; Palasantzas, 2004; Persson, 2006). Therefore, during dynamic footwear–surface interactions, the characteristics of the surface profile will undoubtedly affect the friction (or traction) force developed.

During a horizontal sliding event the asperities of the solid substrate cause cyclic elastic deformation of the viscoelastic rubber material. Internal damping causes energy dissipation during the loading and unloading cycle (Persson, 2001; Palasantzas, 2004; Persson *et al.*, 2002). This loss is the hysteretic component of the contributing friction mechanisms. If local stresses deform the rubber beyond its elastic limit, it will be unable to recover and this results in the tearing of the material leading to additional traction forces at the interface between rubber and surface. Tearing can result in wear and cause the separation of fragments of material from the rubber; this mechanism is termed abrasive wear. The build-up of rubber fragments between the shoe and surface can then affect the friction further by acting as a dry lubrication layer.

Adhesion is the process of junctions forming, due to van der Waals' interaction between the contacting surfaces and the arising friction force is the force required for the junctions to shear. Adhesive friction is more prevalent when rubber slides over a smooth surface and depends significantly on the real contact area (contact between asperities) and therefore the roughness characteristics of the surface the rubber is sliding relative to. On increasingly rough surfaces the contribution of the adhesive component of traction has been found to decrease caused by a reduction in asperity interaction (Palasantzas, 2004; Persson, 2006). An initial decrease in friction/traction coefficient with increasing normal force has been observed with interactions between rubber and hard surfaces, with it becoming constant at higher loads (Persson, 1998). A power relationship was observed between normal force and friction coefficient by Clarke *et al.* (2012) with shoe–surface interactions in tennis. Persson (1998) states that such a relationship will be due to molecular adhesion. As the normal force increases the coefficient of friction (COF) becomes constant as the real area of contact increases proportionally with the normal force.

Persson (1998, 2001) explains how real contact area will be dependent on the wavelength (λ) and amplitude (h) of the surface profile, as well as the loading conditions. Figure 6.5 (adapted from Persson, 1998) illustrates how as the amplitude of the surface roughness is decreased, under the same loading conditions, surface contact will increase. The compressibility of a viscoelastic material leads to its area in contact with a surface of the same profile being dependent on the normal loading conditions. As normal force increases the rubber compresses against the surface increasing asperity contact, as illustrated in Figure 6.5c). Therefore, increased normal force results in greater asperity contact and an increase in the adhesional and hysteretic components of traction.

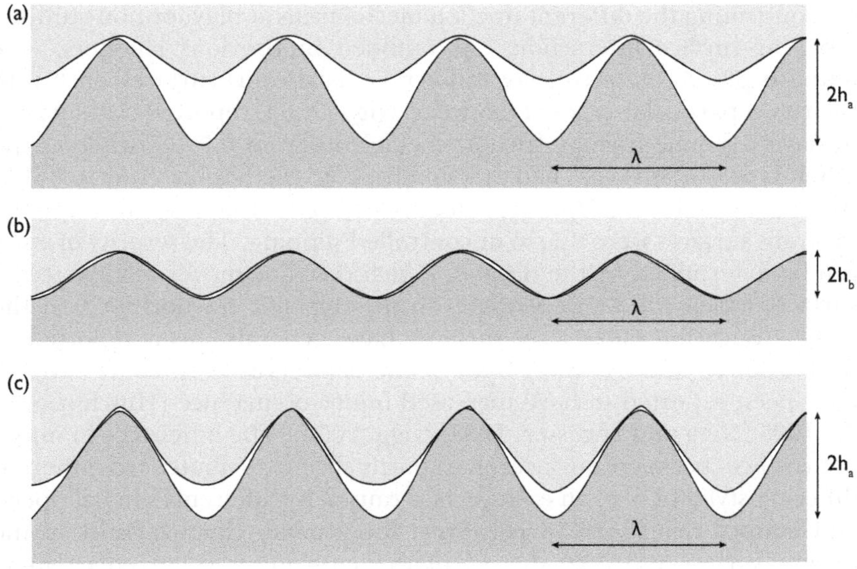


*Figure 6.5* Rubber-surface contacts under applied pressure. (a) The rough surface profile prevents the rubber from completely contacting the surface; (b) Under same pressure as (a), the reduced surface roughness amplitude (h) now allows increased contact between the two surfaces; (c) Same roughness profile as (a), but now increased pressure causes increased contact between the two surfaces. Adapted from Persson (1998).

Clarke *et al.* (2012) highlighted the importance of testing under a range of normal loads as the relationship between normal force and traction force is shoe–surface dependent. This was attributed to changes in the tribological interaction under varying load. In a number of previous studies conducting comparative investigations into sport shoe–surface traction via mechanical test methods the applied normal force has remained at the same value throughout testing (Valiant, 1990; Wojcieszak *et al.*, 1997; Shorten *et al.*, 2003; Williams and Neugebauer, 2007; Wannop *et al.*, 2010). However, this may give misleading results as the relationship between traction force and normal force is dependent on the specific shoe–surface combination. A cross-over point can occur after which shoe–surface combinations will give comparatively different traction measurements. It is therefore potentially misleading to draw conclusions on the traction a player is likely to experience from shoe–surface combinations when based on the mechanical traction value performed under a single normal force.

### *Shoe–surface interactions in tennis*

Tennis is played on a variety of surfaces and is a useful sport for demonstrating the different traction mechanisms at play for non-studded footwear–surface interactions. As outlined in previous chapters, elite tennis is played on grass, clay and acrylic hard-court surfaces, each with their own particular types of footwear. Nigg (2003) reported clay surfaces to have dynamic traction/friction coefficients from 0.5–0.7 whereas the other types of surfaces had traction/friction coefficients from 0.8–1.2. Biener and Caluori (1977) reported 21 per cent of injuries over a range of tennis surfaces were due to uncontrolled slipping. The severity of a slip can be determined by the distance which the shoe moves relative to the surface, which will be dependent on the dynamic traction force at the shoe–surface interface. Clay surfaces have generally been reported to have a lower occurrence of injury, whereas acrylic hard-court surfaces have been reported to have increased injury occurrence (Hutchinson *et al.*, 1995; Nigg and Segesser, 1988; Nigg, 2003). The difference in injury occurrence between surfaces has partly been attributed to inherent differing styles of play on each surface caused by differences in ball speed and bounce (Nigg, 2003). However, the traction characteristics of the playing surface also affect the risk of accidental injury occurrence (Dixon *et al.*, 1999). This has led to the hypothesis accepted by many that surfaces which do not allow controlled sliding movements may increase the potential to cause injury.

Damm *et al.* (2011) used a force platform to measure three-dimensional ground reaction forces (GRF) of the leading leg as tennis players performed a side jump movement out of stance (with fixed foot position) on both an acrylic hard court and an artificial clay surface. The mean peak normal GRFs on both surfaces were not found to be significantly different, but surprisingly, the peak horizontal shear force (Fshear) during the impact phase was found to be significantly greater on the clay surface than on the hard court, facilitating sliding for this surface type.

## *Mechanical testing of tennis shoe–surface interactions*

Clarke *et al.* (2013a) investigated hard-court acrylic tennis surface traction and found, via mechanical testing, that the dynamic traction force achieved generally increases with normal loading, as one would expect (see Figure 6.6). However, the trend with roughness under relatively low normal loading conditions (500N) gave a peak dynamic traction at a mid-range roughness value ($R_a$ = approx. 55μm). However, as the normal load increased to 1,000N, a transition occurred causing the traction to dip slightly over a range of roughness, now giving the lowest traction at mid-range roughness (see Figure 6.6). Clarke *et al.* hypothesised the hysteretic friction mechanisms associated with overcoming surface roughness during sliding became increasingly dominant as normal force increases due to increased asperity contact of the viscoelastic tennis shoe sole.

Acrylic hard-court tennis surfaces are constructed with a coating of acrylic paint and silica sand mix. Clarke *et al.* explained that this is likely to give surfaces a profile with a short wavelength surface (due to the

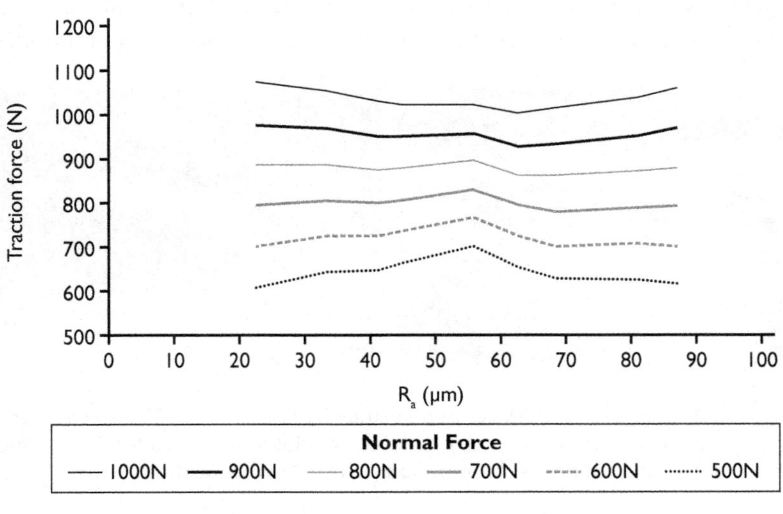


*Figure 6.6* Plot of the traction force against mean average surface roughness ($R_a$) for a range of normal loading conditions on hard-court surface samples. Reproduced from Clarke *et al.* (2013a).

relatively small roughness of the paint layer) overlaid on top of a profile with a longer wavelength (due to the larger-size silica sand particles beneath). As highlighted by Palasantzas (2004) such real surfaces will have a profile with a degree of randomness. The profile characteristics will be dependent on the silica sand particle size and the ratio of paint to sand in the coating mix. When considering surfaces of short- and long-wavelength profiles, Persson (2001) notes that although the applied pressure may be high enough to cause direct contact between the rubber and the surface into the short-wavelength asperities at the top of the surface, it may not be high enough to cause asperity contact within the short-wavelength asperities at the bottom of the long-wavelength profile.

Clarke *et al.* (2013b) also developed a new lab-based test device (see Figure 6.7) to investigate shoe traction on two artificial clay surfaces (one that had a clay infill, one with sand infill) and an acrylic hard court. They found that the infill particle size used in an artificial clay surface will significantly influence the traction developed at the shoe–surface interface. Clay particles can bond in wet and dry conditions, and the initial stiffness and peak traction will depend on the normal force applied to the surface by the shoe, whereas the larger sand particles will exhibit reduced traction caused by a reduction in shear strength. Surfaces with large sand particles will develop lower traction in dry than in wet conditions as the particles are unable to cohere and therefore act as single entities. In dry conditions and under increased normal loading, the traction developed at the shoe–surface interface on an artificial clay surface was found to sometimes be greater than that of the hard-court surface, which illustrates the complex interaction mechanisms that occur.

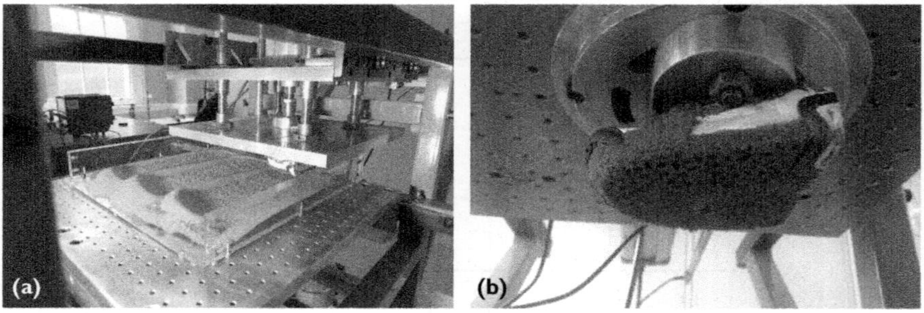


*Figure 6.7* (a) Lab-based test device used in study by Clarke *et al.* (2013b) to investigate tennis shoe traction on clay surfaces; (b) close-up view of forefoot section of tennis shoe in device. Photos: Bob Levene, Intwodimensions.co.uk.

## Final remarks

The findings of studies outlined in this chapter indicate the often complicated interactions that can occur between shoes and surfaces in different sports and play situations. Different friction/traction mechanisms can play a key part in the resulting forces that resist relative movement between shoe and surface, depending on factors such as presence of moisture, shoe/stud penetration and loading, meaning that relative trends for different shoe and surface parameters are not always consistent. This reinforces the fact that mechanical test devices must aim to replicate the relevant forces and velocities that appear in player movements as well as shoe and surface conditions (and therefore the relevant mechanisms), if they are to be used to assess playing performance.

## Key summary points

- The relevant aspects of shoe–surface traction that are to be examined depend largely on the type of movement and sports application (e.g. sprinting in football vs. sliding in tennis). It is also important to consider what the aim of the study is, e.g. injury-reduction, performance-enhancement or a combination of factors.
- There have been a number of studies examining the interaction between studded footwear and different sports surfaces (including artificial and natural turfs). They demonstrate the importance of simulating the relevant aspects of human loading, as appropriate for the aims of the study and practical considerations. Often it is the degree of stud penetration (affected by loading and surface condition) that has a significant effect on the available traction.
- There has been relatively less research activity on non-studded footwear–surface interactions, but it is clear that for non-deformable, solid surfaces such as acrylic tennis hard courts, much knowledge of friction mechanisms from the field of tribology can be applied to better understand the important interactions.

## References

Andersen, T. E., Larsen, O., Tenga, A., Engebretsen, L. and Bahr, R. (2003) 'Football incident analysis: A new video based method to describe injury mechanisms in professional football', *British Journal of Sports Medicine*, 37(3): 226–232.

Arnason, A., Sigurdsson, S. B., Gudmundsson, A., Holme, I., Engebretsen, L. and Bahr, R. (2004) 'Risk factors for injuries in football', *American Journal of Sports Medicine*, 32(1 suppl): 5S–16S.

Baker, S. W. (1990) 'Standards for the playing quality of artificial turf for association football', in R. C. Schmidt, E. M. Milner, and C. A. Morehouse (eds) *Natural and*

*Artificial Playing Fields: Characteristics and Safety Features*. Philadelphia, PA: American Society for Testing and Materials, pp. 48–60. Available at: www.astm.org/DIGITAL_LIBRARY/STP/SOURCE_PAGES/STP1073_foreword.pdf

Baker, S. W. (1991) 'Temporal variation of selected mechanical properties of natural turf football pitches', *Journal of the Sports Turf Research Institute*, 67: 83–92.

Biener, K. and Caluori, P. (1977) 'Tennissportunfälle (tennis injuries)', *Medizinische Klinik*, 72: 754–757.

Canaway, P. M., Bell, M. J., Holmes, G. and Baker, S. W. (1990) 'Standards for the playing quality of natural turf for association football', in R. C. Schmidt, E. M. Milner, and C. A. Morehouse (eds) *Natural and Artificial Playing Fields: Characteristics and Safety Features*. Philadelphia, PA: American Society for Testing and Materials, pp. 29–47. Available at: www.astm.org/DIGITAL_LIBRARY/STP/SOURCE_PAGES/STP1073_foreword.pdf

Canaway, P. and Baker, S. (1993) 'Soil and turf properties governing playing quality', *International Turfgrass Society Research Journal*, 7: 192–200.

Clarke, J. D. (2011) 'Understanding the performance and comfort of soccer boots', PhD thesis, University of Sheffield, UK.

Clarke, J. D., Damm, L., Dixon, S. and Carré, M. J. (2012) 'Understanding the influence of surface roughness on the tribological interactions at the shoe–surface interface in tennis', *Proceedings of the Institution of Mechanical Engineers Part J: Engineering Tribology*, 226(7): 636–647.

Clarke, J. D., Damm, L., Dixon, S. and Carré, M. J. (2013a) 'The effect of normal load force and roughness on the dynamic traction developed at the shoe–surface interface in tennis', *Sports Engineering*, 16: 165–171.

Clarke, J. D., Carré, M. J., Damm, L. and Dixon, S. (2013b) 'The development of an apparatus to understand the traction developed at the shoe–surface interface in tennis', *Proceedings of the Institution of Mechanical Engineers Part P: Journal of Sports Engineering and Technology*, 227(3): 149–160.

Damm, L., Low, D., Richardson, A., Carré, M. J. and Dixon, S. (2011) 'Modulation of tennis players' frictional demand according to surface traction characteristics', Proceedings of the International Society of Biomechanics Congress XXIII, Brussels, Belgium, 3–7 July 2011.

Dixon, S. J., Batt, M. E. and Collop, A. C. (1999) 'Artificial playing surfaces research: A review of medical, engineering and biomechanical aspects', *International Journal of Sports Medicine*, 20(4): 209–218.

Durá, J. V. (1999) 'The influence of friction on sports surfaces in turning movements;', *ISSS Publications* [online]. Available at: www.isss.de/conferences/Mallorca1999/forum5.html (accessed 8 April 2014).

Frederick, E. C. (1986) 'Kinematically mediated effects of sport shoe design: A review', *Journal of Sports Sciences*, 4: 169–184.

González, J. C., Martínez, A., Montero, J., Alemany, S. and Gámez, J. (2003) 'Analysis of the horizontal forces in soccer boot studs for specific movements', Proceedings of the 6th Symposium of the ISB Technical Group on Footwear Biomechanics Conference, Queenstown, New Zealand.

Griffin, L. Y., Albohm, M. J., Arendt, E. A., Bahr, R., Beynnon, B. D., DeMaio, M., Dick, R. W. *et al.* (2006) 'Understanding and preventing noncontact anterior cruciate ligament injuries – A review of the Hunt Valley II meeting', *American Journal of Sports Medicine*, 34(9): 1512–1532.

Gronqvist, R., Hirvonen, M., Rajamaki, E. and Matz, S. (2003) 'The validity and reliability of a portable slip meter for determining floor slipperiness during simulated heel strike', *Accident Analysis and Prevention*, 35(2): 211–225.

Grund, T. and Senner, V. (2010) 'Traction behavior of soccer shoe stud designs under different game-relevant loading conditions', *Procedia Engineering*, 2(2): 2783–2788.

Grund, T., Senner, V. and Gruber, K. (2007) 'Development of a test device for testing soccer boots under game-relevant high-risk loading conditions', *Sports Engineering*, 10(1): 55–63.

Guisasola, I., James, I., Llewellyn, C., Stiles, V. and Dixon, S. (2009) 'Quasi-static mechanical behaviour of soils used for natural turf sports surfaces and stud force prediction', *Sports Engineering*, 12(2): 99–109.

Hutchison, M. R., Laprade, R. F., Burnett, Q. M., Moss, R. and Terpstra, J. (1995) 'Injury surveillance at the USTA Boys' Tennis Championships: A 6-yr study', *Medicine and Science in Sports and Exercise*, 27(6): 826–830.

Lambson, R. B., Barnhill, B. S. and Higgins, R. W. (1996) 'Football cleat design and its effect on anterior cruciate ligament injuries: A three-year prospective study', *American Journal of Sports Medicine*, 24(2): 155–159.

Livesay, G. A., Reda, D. R. and Nauman, E. A. (2006) 'Peak torque and rotational stiffness developed at the shoe–surface interface: The effect of shoe type and playing surface', *American Journal of Sports Medicine*, 34(3): 415–422.

Meyers, M. C. and Barnhill, B. S. (2004) 'Incidence, causes, and severity of high school football injuries on FieldTurf versus natural grass: A 5-year prospective study', *American Journal of Sports Medicine*, 32(7): 1626–1638.

Milburn, P. D. and Barry, E. B. (1998) 'Shoe–surface interaction and the reduction of injury in rugby union', *Sports Medicine*, 25(5): 319–327.

Murphy, D. F., Connolly, D.A.J. and Beynnon, B. D. (2003) 'Risk factors for lower extremity injury: A review of the literature', *British Journal of Sports Medicine*, 37(1): 13–29.

Nigg, B. (2003) 'Injury and performance on tennis surfaces. The effect of tennis surfaces on the game of tennis' [online]. Available at: http://es.hartru.com.planitapps.com/uploads/downloads/Doc_7.pdf (accessed 26 September 2012).

Nigg, B. M. and Segesser, B. (1988) 'The influence of playing surfaces on the load on the locomotor system and on football and tennis injuries', *Sports Medicine*, 5(6): 375–385.

Orchard, J. (2001) 'The AFL penetrometer study: Work in progress', *Journal of Science and Medicine in Sport*, 4(2): 220–232.

Orchard, J. (2002) 'Is there a relationship between ground and climatic conditions and injuries in football?', *Sports Medicine*, 32(7): 419–432.

Orchard, J., Seward, H., McGivern, J. and Hood, S. (1999) 'Rainfall, evaporation and the risk of non-contact anterior cruciate ligament injury in the Australian Football League', *The Medical Journal of Australia*, 170: 304–306.

Palasantzas, G. (2004) 'Influence of self-affine roughness on the adhesive friction coefficient of a rubber body sliding on a solid substrate', *Surface Science*, 565(2–3): 191–196.

Persson, B.N.J. (1998) 'On the theory of rubber friction', *Surface Science*, 401(3): 445–454.

Persson, B.N.J. (2001) 'Theory of rubber friction and contact mechanics', *Journal of Chemical Physics*, 115(8): 3840–3861.

Persson, B.N.J. (2006) 'Rubber friction: Role of the flash temperature', *Journal of Physics: Condensed Matter*, 18(32): 77–89.

Persson, B.N.J., Bucher, F. and Chiaia, B. (2002) 'Elastic contact between randomly rough surfaces: Comparison of theory with numerical results', *Physical Review*, 65(18): 184106.

Powell, J. W. and Schootman, M. (1992) 'A multivariate risk analysis of selected playing surfaces in the national football league: 1980 to 1989: An epidemiologic study of knee injuries', *American Journal of Sports Medicine*, 20(6): 686–694.

Rosa, D., Sanchis, J., Gamez, J., and Alcantara, E. (2007) 'Study on the effect of maintenance operations and season on the traction of natural grass pitches' in P. Fleming (ed.) *STARRS 2007, Proceedings of the Science, Technology and Research into Sport Surfaces Conference*. Loughborough University, UK.

Severn, K. A., Fleming, P. F., Clarke, J. D. and Carré, M. J. (2011) 'Science of synthetic turf surfaces: Investigating traction behaviour', *Proceedings of the Institution of Mechanical Engineers, Part P: Journal of Sports Engineering and Technology*, 225(3): 147–158.

Shorten, M., Hudson, B. and Himmelsbach, J. (2003) 'Shoe–surface traction of conventional and in-filled synthetic turf football surfaces', XIX International Congress on Biomechanics, New Zealand.

Vachon, F. (2004) 'Football boot sole configurations and their influence upon surface adhesion', *ISSS Publications* [online]. Available at: www.isss.de/publications/ArtificialTurf/Vachon%20Friction.pdf (accessed 8 April 2014).

Valiant, G. A. (1990) 'Traction characteristics of outsoles for use on artificial playing surfaces', in R. C. Schmidt, E. M. Milner, and C. A. Morehouse (eds) *Natural and Artificial Playing Fields: Characteristics and Safety Features*. Philadelphia, PA: American Society for Testing and Materials, pp. 61–68. Available at: www.astm.org/DIGITAL_LIBRARY/STP/SOURCE_PAGES/STP1073_foreword.pdf

Volpi, P. (2008) 'Epidemiology and risk factors in soccer', *Medicina Dello Sport*, 61(2): 111–119.

Wannop, J. W., Worobets, J. T. and Stefanyshyn, D. J. (2010) 'Footwear traction and lower extremity joint loading', *American Journal of Sports Medicine*, 38(6): 1221–1228.

Williams, K. R. and Neugebauer, J. M. (2007) 'Ground reaction forces and traction in golf shoes', Proceedings of the 8th Footwear Biomechanics Symposium, Taipei, Taiwan.

Wojcieszak, C., Peixing, J. and Frederick, E. C. (1997) 'A comparison of two friction measuring methods', Proceedings of the 3rd Symposium on Footwear Biomechanics, Tokyo, Japan.

Chapter 7

# Human–shoe–surface interaction

*Loïc Damm, Victoria Stiles and Sharon Dixon*

## Introduction

The present chapter focuses on understanding the complex interaction between humans, shoes and surfaces. Clarifying the relation between mechanical characteristics of shoes and surfaces, and their biomechanical consequences is crucial to improve performance and comfort while maintaining a low risk of injury. A description of shoes is first provided, since their characteristics can vary according to the sport they are dedicated to and can influence interaction with the surface. The requirement for biomechanical (human) tests is highlighted in relation to isolated shoe–surface testing. The chapter then reviews the current status regarding research on the influence of shoe–surface properties on biomechanics in sports.

## Shoe and surface characteristics

### *Sports footwear – key features*

Running is the movement generally considered primarily in the design of a sports shoe. However sport-specific shoes, notably those dedicated to ball games, have to meet the requirements of a broader spectrum of movements including sideward movements like shuffling, twisting and turning. The cushioning and friction properties of shoes must also be suitable for their specific surface of use. The purpose of this section is to describe the structure and characteristics most commonly adopted by footwear manufacturers (Figure 7.1).

The *uppers* (Figure 7.1a) are essential for both comfort and control. To meet the first requirement, mesh ensures good breathability and foam prevents areas of high localised pressure. A tight fit is the prerequisite for good control, this being ensured by specific overlays that link the foot bed to the eyelets of the laces. The tongue includes a layer of foam that transfers the pressure from the laces to a large area. The pattern of shoe

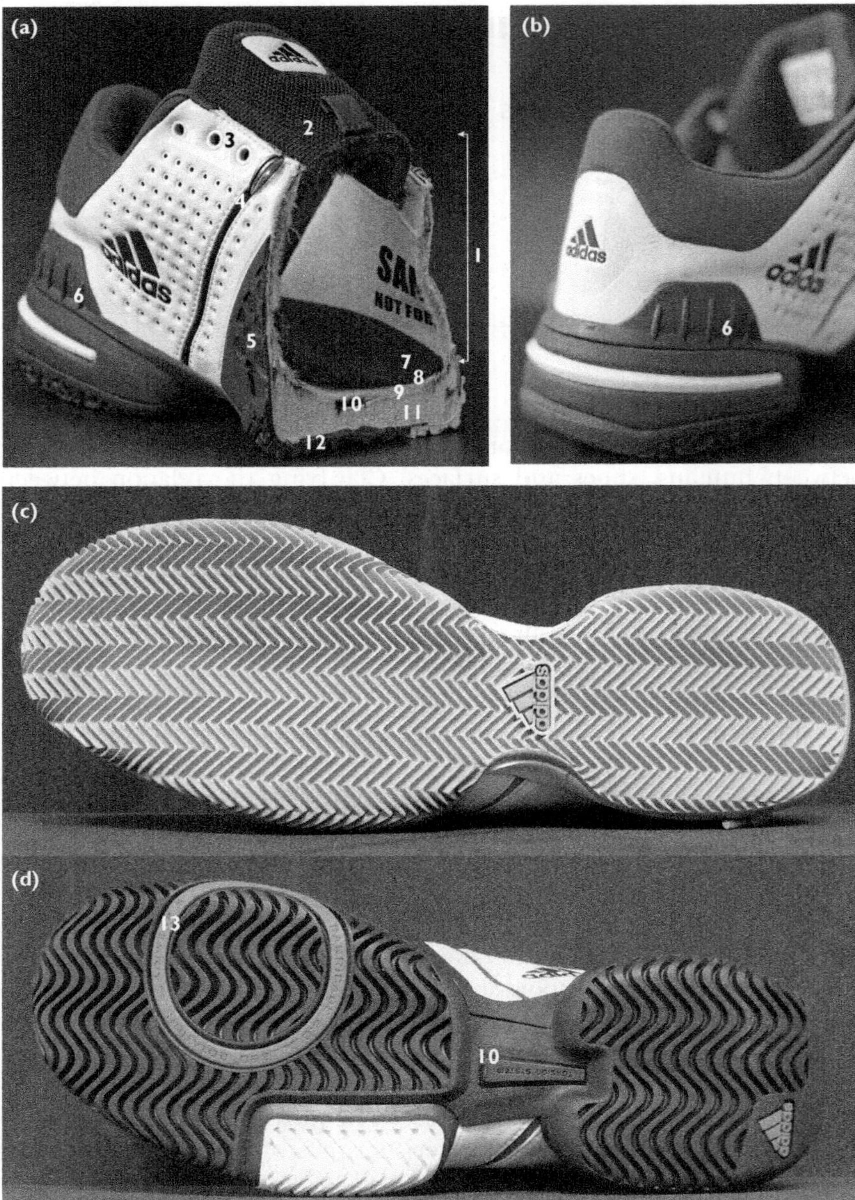


*Figure 7.1* (a) Tennis shoe structure visible after a frontal cut; (b) Detail of heel counter; (c) and (d) Outsole patterns: clay shoes (c) and hard-court shoes (d). 1: uppers; 2: tongue; 3: eyelets; 4: overlay; 5: aeration; 6: heel counter; 7: insole (laminated soft fabric); 8: insole (foam); 9: foot bed; 10: insole board; 11: midsole; 12: outsole; 13: pivot point.

lacing can have an effect on both foot-to-shoe-coupling and comfort (Hagen *et al.*, 2010).

The *heel counter* (Figure 7.1b) is the most rigid part of the upper, aiming to lock the heel in a stable position so that the heel fat pad can interact directly with the cushioning materials of the shoe heel at impact. Its rigidity has also been found to be crucial for control (Van Gheluwe *et al.*, 1999).

The shoe *insole* consists of a removable thin layer moulded on the foot bed. It may include a few millimetres of foam (EVA – ethylene vinyl acetate, rubber, latex), and can have a significant cushioning effect (Windle *et al.*, 1999; Shiba *et al.*, 1995). Insoles are typically covered with laminated soft fabric that optimises friction with the sock, preventing foot sliding (Easterling, 1993).

The *midsole* is commonly filled with polymeric foam, most commonly EVA and polyurethane (for a comparison, see Indesteege *et al.* (1998)). EVA is lighter and polyurethane more durable. These materials are sometimes combined in the same midsole, with the higher density of polyurethane foam being more appropriate in areas of the shoes where good support is required. Other systems utilise the damping and elasticity of large air-filled compartments (e.g. Nike 'air') or specific gels (e.g. Ascis gel). Despite the diversity of designs, the rationale is the same, i.e. providing cushioning characteristics to the midsole. The distribution of impact absorbing material varies according to the function of the shoe. For example, running shoes classically have their thickest cushioning material layer at the heel: in heel-toe running, the impact represents most of the input energy and the rate of energy dissipation during the subsequent forefoot contact is much lower (Shorten, 1993). In ball sports, where foot position at landing is variable, a full-length cushioned midsole has been suggested to be desirable (McPoil, 2000).

The *insole board* influences the coupling between the rearfoot and forefoot. Eversion/inversion of the forefoot relative to the rearfoot has been described as 'torsion' (Stacoff *et al.*, 1989). During the stance phase, torsion of the foot allows the forefoot to conform to the geometry of the surface without constraining the position of the rearfoot. Kälin *et al.* (1989) showed that when running a curve barefoot, the forefoot adjusts to the floor without forcing the rearfoot into excessive inversion. Generally, shoes would reduce the natural torsion relative to barefoot running (Stacoff *et al.*, 1991; Morio *et al.*, 2009). Balancing the requirements for rearfoot support to prevent overpronation during the loading phase, while providing low torsional stiffness to prevent mechanical coupling between the forefoot and rearfoot, is technically challenging. Board lasting, where a moulded stiff polyurethane bar is part of the midsole, aims to support the midfoot while permitting torsion between the rear and forefoot (Craton and McKenzie, 1993; Michel *et al.*, 2009).

*Outsoles* (Figure 7.1c, d) are typically constructed from polyurethane rubbers due to their resistance to abrasion. The tread pattern compensates for the relatively low friction level of polyurethane when it is wet (Bartlett, 1999). This tread pattern is surface-specific. For example, in tennis, a sport where participation takes place on many different types of surface, there are marked differences in shoe outsole tread. The sole of shoes designed for play on carpet are usually relatively smooth. If this type of shoe were used on clay, the outsole would interact with the easily movable top particles of clay and would provide negligible grip. On this latter surface, classical herring-bone patterns allow the clay to enter the grooves so that the contours of the outsole penetrate the superficial layer of the surface. Studs (cleats) are added to the outsole for sports played on surfaces such as natural turf, to provide traction between the shoe and surface.

In recent years an increased interest in barefoot running has lead manufacturers to design *minimal shoes*. The most radical ones are similar to gloves and do not include any cushioning or rigid material, but simply a soft and flexible material that is designed to provide protection against the rough ground surface. The toebox is wide and extensible to allow the toes to spread apart and there is no arch support. There is no connection between the forefoot and the rearfoot, and no motion control effect – aiming to replicate foot movement when running barefoot (Squadrone and Gallozzi, 2009).

## Properties of sports shoes and surfaces

Providing appropriate friction and cushioning are the basic requirements of the shoe–surface combination. The properties of materials used in the construction of sports shoes and surfaces are most typically tested in isolation. Properties for the characterisation of sports surfaces have been outlined in detail in Chapter 3. Properties for the characterisation of shoes in isolation and shoe–surface combinations are described below.

### Cushioning

The term cushioning has been used to refer to the hardness of footwear materials, their stiffness or their ability to reduce impact forces. Durometers provide a measure of material ('Shore') hardness: a typical test comprises pressing a standardised foot onto the material with a given force; the elastic deflection of the material can be read, the greater it is, the lower the hardness (Mills, 2007). According to Nike's US patent 4535553 (1983), the Shore A hardness test value should be >25 in foams used in midsoles. The Young's modulus, defined as the ratio of tensile stress over the tensile strain in the linear portion of the stress-strain curve, gives a measure of stiffness of elastic materials. Due to the non linear response of shoe foams to compression and the complex structure of the polymer that creates a complex strain field under the indenter, the Young's modulus is not sufficient to describe hardness (Mills, 2007). A standard drop test procedure has been developed to quantify the impact attenuation properties of footwear by measuring the deceleration of a mass during impact with the shoe (ASTM F1976-06). Each of these described shoe properties focus on measuring the shoe in isolation, with no consideration of the human interacting with the shoe, or the surface on which the shoe will be worn. In addition, the loading in each of the described test procedures is applied normal to the tested material surface. This is not representative of typical loading in sports and also does not account for the anisotropic behaviour of the loaded materials.

### *Friction*

Shoe friction cannot be measured in isolation – this property depends on the interaction between the shoe and surface. The resultant force acting between the shoe outsole and the surface can be resolved into two components: the normal component and the tangential one. The tangential force, termed friction force, determines whether the contacting surfaces can move relative to one another. The theoretical description of friction defines the coefficient of friction as the ratio of the normal ($F_n$) and shear/friction ($F_f$) components of the force. The coefficient of static friction $\mu_s$ (Equation 7.1) is used to calculate the force that needs to be overcome to initiate movement between the two contacting bodies, whereas the coefficient of dynamic friction $\mu_d$ (Equation 7.2) is necessary to calculate the friction force once the movement has started.

$$F_f < \mu_s F_n \qquad \text{(Equation 7.1)}$$

$$F_f = \mu_d F_n \qquad \text{(Equation 7.2)}$$

Equation 7.2 is Amonton's or Coulomb's Law, and from it, it appears that friction is directly proportional to the load. Perhaps surprising is the absence of the contact area in the formula. This point can be accounted for if we consider that contact area depends on the load: when it increases, so does the contact area. However, study of the behaviour of the shoe–surface interaction has demonstrated that while these laws are suitable to describe the interaction between uniform rigid surfaces, they fail to predict the behaviour of interactions between compliant and resilient materials such as footwear and sports surfaces (James, 1980; Valiant, 1987, 1990). As described in Chapter 6, the interaction between the shoe and surface also varies with normal loading, pressure, contact area and sliding velocity.

In addition to translational friction that affects running, landing or stopping movements, rotational friction is a determinant during foot rotation. Rotational friction follows the same physical rules as translational friction: when rotating the foot, low rotational friction is desirable for fast and safe rotations. This has influenced outsole construction of sports shoes – for example, many manufacturers of tennis shoes have added a circular pattern on the medial part of the forefoot (Figure 7.1d, Label 13).

## Biomechanical testing of shoe–surface properties

### *Experimental approaches*

Ground reaction force (GRF) data obtained from a force plate provide the resultant force vector and its location on the force plate surface. Typical force profiles for sports movements are presented in Figure 7.2. The acceleration of the centre of mass determines these loading and unloading phases. The plot of the vertical force during heel-toe running (Figure 7.2a) typically exhibits two peaks. The first high-frequency (10–15Hz) one predominantly reflects the impact forces during initial foot–ground contact. The second low-frequency (1–3Hz) one is representative of active forces (Nigg, 1983). Variables commonly reported in studies are maximum amplitude for both impact and active forces, and the maximal slope of the vertical force curve during the 50ms following foot strike, also referred to as maximum loading rate.

While force plate data are relatively easy to obtain for different sports movements, the measure of GRF does have some limitations. The magnitude of GRF relates to the acceleration of the total body mass, and does not directly indicate the force acting on the foot nor the distribution of force. In contrast, the availability of pressure measuring systems allows the direct measurement of the distribution of force across the shoe outsole surface or shoe–foot interface, depending on whether a plate or an insole system is used. Pressure measurement with insoles provides a map of pressure distribution across the plantar surface of the foot, revealing the regions of high pressure (Figure 7.2 and 7.3b). Pressure insoles have the additional benefit of acquiring data from multiple steps, without putting any constraints on foot location, removing virtually any constraint on the type of movement investigated (Cavanagh *et al.*, 1992).

Kinematics refers to the branch of biomechanics that describes the motion of the body or its segments without consideration of the causes of motion, i.e. forces. Experimental techniques used to collect kinematic variables include:

1 Goniometers to measure joint angles.
2 Accelerometers to measure segmental accelerations.

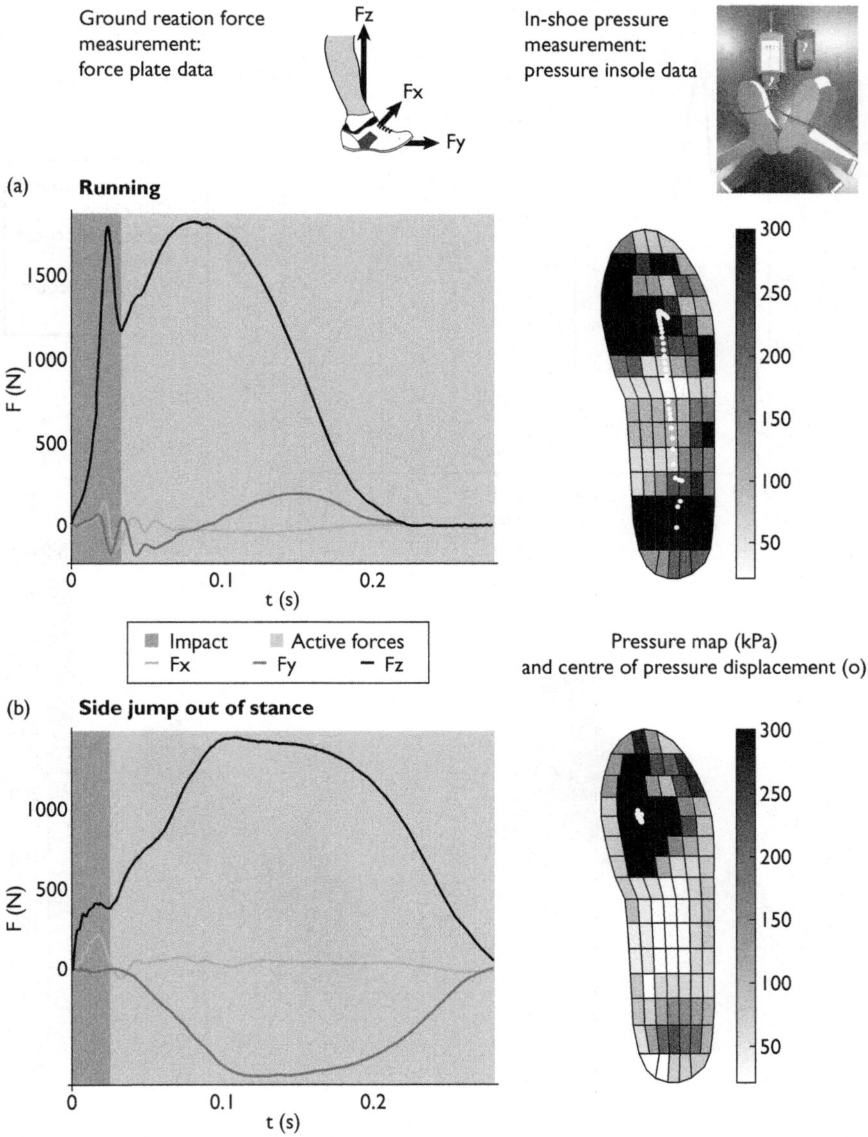


*Figure 7.2* GRF and pressure map during running (a) and side jump out of stance (b).

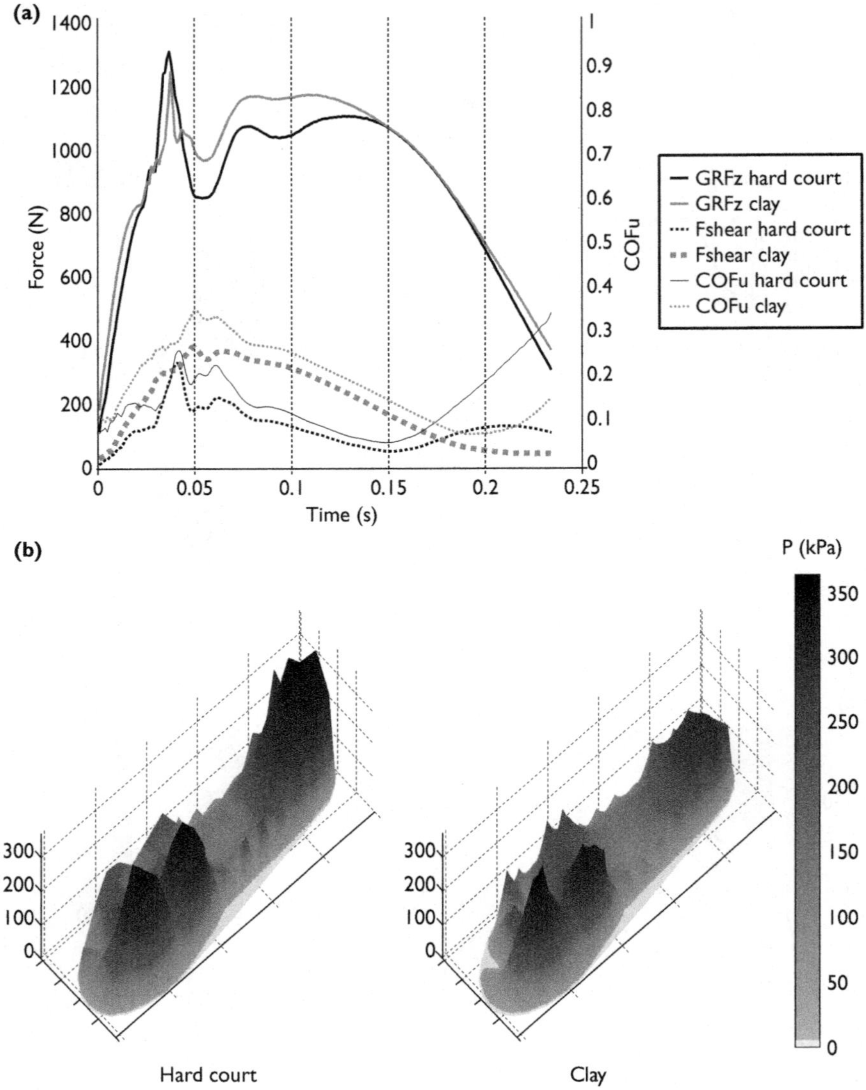


*Figure 7.3* (a) Example of the vertical component of GRF (GRFz), shear force (Fshear), and utilised coefficient of friction (COFu) for one subject during a tennis open-stance running forehand; (b) Map of maximal pressure recorded during running forehand on hard court and clay for one subject.

3 Video-based systems combined with digitising.
4 3D motion-capture systems to directly measure the position of markers placed on the body.

3D motion-capture systems (passive marker systems such as Oqus cameras from Qualisys (Qualisys AB, Sweden) and Vicon (Vicon Motion Systems Ltd, UK), or active markers systems like Codamotion (Charnwood Dynamics Ltd, UK)) are the technique of choice because, from the position of specific markers, body segment position and orientation are directly calculated, and the calculation of joint angles, and their time derivatives, velocity and acceleration, is also straightforward (Kwon, 2008).

Lightweight accelerometers directly strapped to the skin can measure the acceleration of specific body segments: this technique is complementary to force plate data collection, because it gives access to the reconstruction of segmental inertia and can measure the shock transmission throughout the body (Nigg *et al.*, 1995).

When one leg supports the body, as is the case during many sports movements, synchronised GRF and kinematics can be combined with segmental inertial characteristics as input variables to compute joint forces and torques following d'Alembert's principle (Hof, 1992): estimation of forces in internal structures is achieved using the inverse dynamics approach. The quality of the results depends on the initial assumptions of the model, the mathematical methods used and the quality of the kinematic and kinetic data collected (Herzog and Leonard, 1991).

### Modelling approaches

During foot impact with the ground each body segment accelerates with its own direction and rate (Shorten, 2002), contributing to the resultant ground reaction force. An approach developed to capture the specific contribution of the different parts of the kinematic chain is modelling. An extreme simplification that can nevertheless provide realistic simulation, is represented by the effective mass model, where the effective mass is the specific mass that collides with the ground and is decelerated to produce the impact force (Nigg, 2010). The effective mass depends on leg geometry and leg stiffness (Denoth, 1986).

Spring-mass or spring-damper-mass models are commonly used to simulate GRF during locomotion (Alexander, 1988; Cavagna *et al.*, 1988; McMahon and Cheng, 1990; Thompson and Raibert, 1990; Ferris *et al.*, 1999; Nikooyan and Zadpoor, 2011). Alexander (1988), cited in Nigg (2010), demonstrated how different combinations of masses, springs and dampers produce force profiles of different shape, for example a parabolic curve by a simple mass-spring system with the spring contacting the ground, compared with a double mass system connected with a spring, producing a biphasic curve. Such models are representative of the human body, with different masses that decelerate at their own rate at impact, determining the different components of the GRF. These models can be manipulated to produce GRF profiles and to investigate the effect of varying the model components.

In order to simulate the coupling between soft and rigid tissues of the human body, models incorporating non-rigid masses, called 'wobbling masses', have been developed. Nigg and Liu (1999) describe a sophisticated model where masses, spring constant and damping coefficients can be varied to match the mechanical characteristics of the specific elements of the human body and the shoe–surface combination. Investigation of the influence of the shoe–surface interface using this approach revealed that the mechanical properties of the shoe or the ground were a dominant factor in determining the predicted loading rate.

The characterisation of footwear and shoe–surface properties has been detailed, and biomechanical experimental and modelling approaches have been identified. We will now evaluate the current status regarding understanding of the influence of cushioning ability and friction properties on human biomechanics.

## Evidence from biomechanical testing of the shoe–surface combination

Approaches to mechanical testing of sports surfaces have been described in Chapter 3 and some of the limitations of such tests have been identified. In particular, while the described tests are useful for ranking of surfaces, relating the results to human biomechanics is a challenge if the specific material combinations occurring during human performance have not been replicated. This has influenced the inability of mechanical testing to reliably predict biomechanical behaviour for specific shoe–surface combinations. In addition, mechanical tests typically do not replicate the loading patterns applied during human interaction with the surface. Firstly, the magnitudes of load provided by mechanical and biomechanical tests can appear very different. For example, the typical contact pressures measured with the Artificial Athlete Berlin vary from 700kPa on synthetic turf to 1,500kPa on macadam (Young and Fleming, 2007). On grass and asphalt, measures from pressure insoles did not show values higher than 350kPa (Tessutti *et al.*, 2010). Secondly, the loading patterns occurring during human interaction are not simulated adequately by the majority of mechanical test devices. Loading during human–shoe–surface interaction in heel-strike running, for example, is influenced by rapid plantar flexion and rearfoot pronation after footstrike, (Nilsson *et al.*, 1985; Nigg *et al.*, 1987; Perry and Lafortune, 1995), which is not represented by a typical mechanical test device.

As suggested by Dixon *et al.* (1999), the most appropriate approach for friction testing is the development of standardised tests using typical shoe sole material. As outlined in Chapters 3 and 6, ideally biomechanical data should be used to determine the specific loading conditions occurring during sports performance to develop representative mechanical test devices that contact the surface at specific angles and magnitudes of velocity (Dixon and Cooke, 2004). Such a test is described in Chapter 6 and in Clarke *et al.* (2012).

In Chapters 3 and 6, the mechanical properties of surfaces and the mechanical tests used to measure these have been described. The following sub-sections evaluate the current status regarding understanding of the influence of changes in sports surface cushioning and friction properties on the biomechanics of human movement in sports.

### Effects of shoe and surface cushioning

Cushioning materials have been included in shoes in an effort to reduce impact forces associated with initial ground impact, on the assumption that these are associated with the development of injuries (see Chapter 4). Force plates were initially used to evaluate the shock-absorbing function of shoes. Studies done during the early development of shoe cushioning systems did not show any striking effect on the magnitude of impact force (Clarke *et al.*, 1983), while lower loading rates have sometimes been observed (Nigg *et al.*, 1986; Dixon *et al.*, 2008).

There is evidence that force plate data are suitable for the detection of extreme differences in footwear cushioning, such as the higher loading rate frequently reported during barefoot running compared to running in sports shoes (Cole *et al.*, 1995; De Wit *et al.*, 2000). Aerts and De Clercq (1993), applying an impact on a fixed foot–shoe combination observed lower peak loading rates for soft- compared with hard-soled conditions. Similarly, Lafortune *et al.* (1996), using a human pendulum to deliver controlled impacts to the foot, reported a soft EVA interface to reduce impact compared with a hard EVA foam. These results suggest that for controlled impacts of the lower limb, the impact force is determined by the impact interface (shoe–surface combination), but that this is generally in contrast to the previously described evidence from in-vivo experiments where humans have performed sports movements and forces are quantified with a force plate. In contrast, Dixon and Stiles (2003) demonstrated a greater sensitivity of pressure insoles to the cushioning properties of footwear.

Although studies of sports surfaces have been less widespread than those of sports shoe cushioning, the conflicting results regarding the effects of shoe cushioning on human loading have been mirrored in surface testing. When running on surfaces with differing mechanical properties, peak impact forces measured with a force plate have typically been unchanged (Feehery, 1986; Nigg and Yeadon, 1987; Wilson *et al.*, 1997). Dixon *et al.* (2000) also demonstrated no significant differences in magnitude of force for surfaces of different mechanical cushioning. However, a significant reduction in loading rate of peak impact force was detected for the surface with the most mechanical cushioning compared with the least cushioned surface. The greater sensitivity of in-shoe pressure data has also been reported for surface testing, with Dixon *et al.* (2008) recording in-shoe pressure data during heel-toe running on soils of different densities and revealing no significant differences in the peak force or loading rate between surfaces, but a significantly lower heel pressure for the soft surface compared with the hard one. Modelling studies have also revealed different results to those obtained with force plates. Ly *et al.* (2010), utilising a spring-damper-mass model to represent the shoe midsole and the ground in two different layers, found that the ground stiffness greatly affected the force peak and the loading rate.

For studies of shoe and surface cushioning, loading rate of ground reaction force and peak pressure variables have been found to be more sensitive to variation in mechanical cushioning than the peak impact force. If surface and shoe cushioning properties are believed to play a role in injury development, there is a requirement to understand in detail what GRF represents and to identify the specific biomechanical mechanisms that affect the GRF. Approaches that could help to improve understanding in this area are the study of biomechanical adaptation and the frequency analysis of GRF data.

### *Biomechanical Adaptation*

As an interface between the body and the environment, *stiffness* characteristics of the leg ensure a stable coupling between them. We can define the *stiffness* as the amount of force (stress) per unit of deflection (strain) (Hamill and Knutzen, 2008). During contact with the ground, the kinematic chain also absorbs force through joint rotation. The leg, therefore, does not act only as a spring but also as a damping system to decelerate the body momentum. The term *impedance* encompasses inertia, damping and stiffness, and is therefore most appropriate for quantifying this behaviour.

In studies of hopping or jumping an increased leg impedance has been demonstrated on more compliant surfaces (Gollhofer, 1987; McNitt-Gray *et al.*, 1993; McNitt-Gray *et al.*, 1994). Studying specifically the hopping task, Farley *et al.* (1998) showed that leg impedance varies in an inverse proportion to that of the surface, such that the overall system impedance remains constant. These changes in impedance result in the vertical displacement of the centre of mass being unchanged at the transition to a softer or harder surface (Ferris *et al.*, 1998). Thus the observed mechanical changes occurring in the lower limb act to maintain this centre of mass trajectory and thus a consistent overall movement pattern.

One mechanism by which the observed changes in lower limb impedance can occur is through kinematic adaptation. Bobbert *et al.* (1992) attributed impedance adjustment of the lower extremity during impact to the variation of lower extremity geometry of the body immediately before ground contact. Studies focused on hopping have observed that knee contact angle significantly influences both peak ground reaction forces and segment accelerations when landing after a jump (Farley *et al.*, 1998; Farley and Morgenroth, 1999; Hobara *et al.*, 2009; Elvin *et al.*, 2007). During jump landings on different surfaces, accommodation to a more compliant surface has been found to be achieved through reduced knee flexion following landing (Sanders and Allen, 1993). For running, an increased initial knee flexion has been suggested to reduce the lower extremity impedance, compensating for increased stiffness of the surface for some individuals (Dixon *et al.*, 2000). However, inter-subject variability was observed in the kinematic response, consistent with studies of adaptation to shoe cushioning (Azevedo *et al.*, 2005).

In addition to the observed changes in knee kinematics, the potential role of the ankle joint in providing cushioning has also been demonstrated. The contribution of the ankle joint to cushioning during landing from a vertical jump with forefoot contact followed by heel contact has been demonstrated by Brizuela *et al.* (1997). These authors found that restricted ankle dorsi-plantar flexion range through wearing footwear with high ankle support increased the forefoot impact force, thus indirectly demonstrating the role of ankle flexion in providing cushioning of impact force during forefoot landings. In support of this suggestion, when a hopping subject encounters an unpredictable harder surface both knee and ankle flexion angles have been found to participate in the extra necessary damping (Moritz and Farley, 2004).

Greater rearfoot pronation and/or pronation velocity have also been demonstrated to reduce the impact force (Kälin *et al.*, 1985; Luethi *et al.*, 1987; Luethi and Stacoff, 1987), with interventions that increase the subtalar joint moment arm, such as the shoe lateral heel flare, being found to increase initial pronation (Nigg and Morlock, 1987). The role of the surface in influencing rearfoot movement (eversion/pronation) has typically been ignored, but is likely to be crucial. For example, the effect of a large lateral heel flare on a shoe will differ for a soft surface compared with a hard one, highlighting the importance of considering both the shoe and surface in such analyses.

The balance between impact absorption through kinematic adaptation and conservation of energy has been suggested to be a compromise (Hardin *et al.*, 2004). The leg acts to partially absorb the impact and subsequently some energy, with this strategy having a metabolic cost (McMahon *et al.*, 1987). The conversion of kinetic energy into angular motion through segmental rotation lowers the peak force: what makes the leg more compliant is the increase of flexion velocity. As proposed by Wright *et al.* (1997), the increased rate of knee flexion decreases inertia of the effective mass involved in the collision responsible for the impact. These observations call for further investigation of muscle recruitment across different shoe surface conditions: muscular activity influences both energy cost and impedance of the kinematic chain and electromyography (EMG) measurements could indicate how the control of both variables is conciliated.

### *GRF temporal and spatial analysis*

The discrepancy between mechanical test results and modelling studies compared with force plate testing of shoe–surface cushioning can also be explored by analysing vertical GRF spatial and temporal information. Pressure data for heel-strike running have revealed that parts of the forefoot, most typically the fifth metatarsal, are already in contact with the ground at the time of peak impact force (Shorten, 2002). Thus, peak impact force obtained with a force plate does not only represent the 'heel impact'. Pressure insoles allow the measurement of localised load at the heel, rather than the resulting force, explaining the discrepancy between force plate and pressure data when comparing cushioning systems. Figure 7.3 provides some examples of force and pressure data collected during a tennis forehand: while the vertical force measured by the force plate remains similar across surfaces, the pressure maps differ.

Shorten (2002) utilised a spectral analysis and revealed the high-frequency (>= 12Hz) and the low-frequency (<= 8Hz) components of GRF. Interestingly, the impact force magnitude measured on the GRF curve is not only the by-product of the high frequency heel impact but the sum of it with the low-frequency motion of centre of mass of the body. If we keep in mind that active components contribute to the impact force amplitude that we can read on the traditional GRF curve during heel-toe running, the effects of cushioning can be revisited. Shorten and Mientjes (2011) found a correlation between the amplitude of the high-frequency component of the GRF during heel-toe running and shoe cushioning. Softer shoes reduced the high-frequency impact force and also delayed the occurrence of its peak, indicating an effect on loading rate.

The differing conclusions about cushioning between study approaches are therefore likely a result of the interference between cushioning effect and summation of high- and low-frequency components of GRF (Shorten and Mientjes, 2011). Since cushioned shoes or surfaces delay the occurrence of the high-frequency impact peak, it is summed with a higher low-frequency active force, resulting in an apparently higher peak impact force. Human adaptation in kinematics and differences in muscle activity (EMG) may also play a role in the observed discrepancies.

### *Effects of shoe–surface friction*

As previously highlighted, insufficient friction or traction can cause a slip, which will result in a loss of performance, or may lead to unexpected movements or a fall, which may cause injury. Good grip, on the contrary, could contribute to improved performance – better turning ability for example (Alexander, 2002). A good grip may, however, increase injury risk if the foot 'sticks' unexpectedly on the surface, for example to cause an ankle inversion injury. The following sections outline biomechanical evidence regarding shoe–surface friction, considering both performance and injury implications.

#### *Performance*

While insufficient friction may adversely influence performance, and good grip has been associated with improved performance, the number of studies dedicated to investigating the relationship between friction and performance is limited. Specific sports examples illustrate how friction characteristics can dramatically change performance.

For running, Morin *et al.* (2011) suggested that sprint performance is related to the ability to produce high-net positive horizontal force, with the optimisation of performance relying on the orientation of the resultant GRF and not its magnitude. In support of this, a more forward-oriented reaction force has been found to generate higher acceleration (Kugler and Janshen, 2010). While these studies were not dedicated to evaluation of the influence of friction characteristics of surfaces on performance, they indirectly show the interrelation between these variables: powerful propulsive force requires maximising of horizontal forces, which raises the demand for friction. The coefficient of friction should be high enough to allow friction forces that match a runner's demand and subsequently avoid sliding.

Curve running also reveals the influence of friction on performance. Luo and Stefanyshyn (2011a) hypothesised footwear mechanical friction as the limiting factor for maximal curve sprinting speed. They observed sprinters' friction demand and the centre of mass speed when negotiating a curve to increase if the available friction of the shoe–surface combination increases. This effect was only observed up to a coefficient of friction of 0.8, with no improvement for the last tested coefficient of 1.2. For this task, a higher coefficient of friction permits the application of a more horizontally orientated GRF vector, allowing the runner to lean more toward the centre of the curve (Luo and Stefanyshyn, 2011b). This strategy relies on the friction properties of the interacting shoe and surface, although there appear to be other limiting factors for extremely high coefficients of friction above 0.8.

To evaluate performance implications of the traction properties of football shoes for specific playing surfaces, Hennig and Sterzing (2010) designed a functional traction test measuring the time necessary for a participant to complete a task including accelerations, decelerations, slaloms and cutting movements. Using this test, Sterzing *et al.* (2009) showed that variation in studs (cleats) can dramatically affect performance: the task time was improved (decreased) by 26 per cent when wearing the most appropriate shoes for the surface, with longer studs improving functional traction on natural turf. Sterzing *et al.* (2010), using the same functional traction test, demonstrated that a prototype shoe characterised by multiple and low studs evenly distributed across the rearfoot and the forefoot areas achieved better traction performance on artificial turf than traditional studded footwear designed for natural turf. In addition to the optimal stud design being specific to the surface, the condition of the surface is also essential: up to 21 per cent improvement was noted in running times on firm natural grass compared to natural grass covered by ice and snow (Sterzing *et al.*, 2010).

### *Protection against injuries*

While a high level of shoe–surface friction is required for optimum acceleration and changes in direction, it is important that friction is sufficiently low such that loads acting on the body do not exceed thresholds for damage.

Curve running can be used to illustrate the balance between performance and safety. During curve running there is asymmetry of force distribution between legs, the inside leg generating smaller peak forces compared to the outside leg (Chang and Kram, 2007). Since faster sprint speeds correlate with greater peak vertical GRF (Weyand *et al.*, 2000), the inside leg appears to be the factor limiting speed during curve running. The low GRF exerted by the inside leg in curve running could be explained by the frontal plane knee joint moments, believed to provide the required joint stability, reaching their limit. The muscles that stabilise joints in the frontal plane during curve running are likely to reach their limits before the extensors, constraining the ability to increase sagittal plane extension moments and thus apply increased force. A requirement to work within this safe physiological limit could therefore explain why Luo and Stefanyshyn (2011a) did not observe any performance improvement for a friction coefficient above 0.8.

Dura *et al.* (1999) compared the performance of an 180-degree turn for five playing surfaces with different friction properties. While the time taken to change direction on the different surfaces was comparable, the time taken in the braking phase of the turn was highest for surfaces with relatively high coefficients of friction. This allowed time for more knee flexion than that observed for the surfaces with lower friction. The authors suggested that this increase in knee flexion is a protective mechanism against potential high loads that may result from the limited sliding on these surfaces. It was also found that the maximum knee moment during turning was higher on surfaces with higher friction. The authors suggested that humans adapt in an attempt to maintain forces and moment values below acceptable limits.

Sliding between the shoe and surface may be safe, when it is controlled and expected. Calculating joint moments during v-cut movements performed by basketball players on sliding and non-sliding surfaces, Nigg *et al.* (2009) concluded that surfaces that allow a few millimetres of horizontal movement during ground contact may reduce joint loading at the ankle. However, joint loading at the knee was increased. The interlocking tile surfaces that were tested in this study did not offer the dynamic stability of surfaces where sliding often occurs, such as on clay courts used for tennis. On this type of surface, when the horizontal component of the ground reaction force exceeds the maximum friction force, sliding occurs and subsequently limits internal loads. Tennis surfaces provide a good example of how surfaces where players can slide can be safe. Stucke *et al.* (1984) measured GRF and movement patterns during starting, stopping and turning movements on three different surfaces including clay. It was found that when performing a stopping movement on a clay surface, the amount of knee flexion remained reasonably constant throughout the movement, with sliding occurring between the shoe and surface. However, when performing the same task on an artificial sports surface, the high friction resulted in negligible sliding occurring, and knee flexion was found to occur throughout the stopping movement. Similarly, in a recent data collection at the University of Exeter Biomechanics Research Laboratory, during a tennis running forehand movement we observed higher knee flexion on a hard court compared to clay. This knee flexion throughout the braking phase could contribute to smooth braking. Figure 7.3a illustrates the friction demand during a tennis-specific movement showing greater shear force on clay than hard court: tennis players can indeed increase their friction demand on clay to facilitate sliding and decrease it on a high coefficient of friction surface like an acrylic hard court.

Since the ideal coefficient of friction will vary for different applications, and the majority of sports are characterised by a range of different movements and playing surfaces, it is a difficult task to specify the most appropriate friction properties of a shoe–surface combination. However, Dura et *al.* (1999) concluded in their study of turning, that a coefficient of friction of around 0.4 is desirable. This is comparable to that suggested by Nigg and Yeadon (1987), but is in contrast to the value of up to 0.8 indicated by Luo and Stefanyshyn (2011a).

## Final remarks

Overall, this chapter has highlighted how detailed biomechanical studies can improve our understanding of the influence of surface properties on human behaviour beyond what is provided by mechanical tests alone. Biomechanical testing can be used to inform the development of appropriate mechanical test procedures, and can reveal the influence of specific mechanical characteristics on the human performer.

## Key summary points

- Mechanical tests should ideally replicate the materials and loading of specific human–shoe–surface interactions.
- Shoe–surface cushioning does not tend to influence peak impact force because of the limitations of the GRF variable measured with a force plate.
- Increased shoe–surface cushioning can reduce localised loading at the foot plantar surface and the aspects of GRF associated with impact, suggesting a potential influence on injury risk.
- Shoe–surface friction is highly influential on performance, with too high or too low a friction having an adverse effect.
- There is a balance between optimal performance and minimising injury risk with appropriate shoe–surface friction.
- The investigation of joint moments during human movement has suggested that the physiological limits of internal loading influence adaptation to different shoe–surface combinations in sports.

## References

Aerts, P. and De Clercq, D. (1993) 'Deformation characteristics of the heel region of the shod foot during a simulated heel strike: the effect of varying midsole hardness', *Journal of Sports Science*, 11: 449–461.

Alexander, R. M. (1988) *Elastic Mechanisms in Animal Movement*. Cambridge: Cambridge University Press.

Alexander, R. M. (2002) *Principles of Animal Locomotion*. Princeton, NJ: Princeton University Press.

Azevedo, L. B., Schwellnus, M. P., Lambert, M. and Vaughan, C. L. (2005) 'Effect of running shoes on biomechanics and subject variability', 7th Symposium on Footwear Biomechanics, 27–29 July, Cleveland, Ohio.

Bartlett, R. (1999) *Sports Biomechanics: Reducing Injury and Improving Performance*. Abingdon: Spon Press.

Bobbert, M. F., Yeadon, M. R. and Nigg, B. M. (1992) 'Mechanical analysis of the landing phase in heel-toe running', *Journal of Biomechanics*, 25: 223–234.

Brizuela, G., Llana, S., Ferrandis, R. and Garcia-Belenguer, A. C. (1997) 'The influence of basketball shoes with increased ankle support on shock attenuation and performance in running and jumping', *Journal of Sports Science*, 15: 505–515.

Cavagna, G. A., Franzetti, P., Heglund, N. C. and Willems, P. (1988) 'The determinants of the step frequency in running, trotting and hopping in man and other vertebrates', *Journal of Physiology*, 399: 81–92.

Cavanagh, P. R., Hewitt, F. G. and Perry, J. E. (1992) 'In-shoe plantar pressure measurement: A review', *The Foot*, 2: 185–194.

Chang, Y. H. and Kram, R. (2007) 'Limitations to maximum running speed on flat curves', *Journal of Experimental Biology*, 210: 971–982.

Clarke, J., Carré, M., Damm, L. and Dixon, S. (2012) 'The influence of surface characteristics on the tribological interactions at the shoe–surface interface in tennis', *Procedia Engineering*, 34: 866–887, 19th Conference of the International Sports Engineering Association (ISEA), Lowell, MA, USA.

Clarke, T. E., Frederick, E. C. and Cooper, L. B. (1983) 'Effects of shoe cushioning upon ground reaction forces in running', *International Journal of Sports Medicine*, 4: 247–251.

Cole, G. K., Nigg, B. M., Fick, G. H. and Morlock, M. M. (1995) 'Internal loading of the foot and ankle during impact in running', *Journal of Applied Biomechanics*, 11: 25–46.

Craton, N. and McKenzie, D. C. (1993) 'Orthotics in injury prevention', in Renström, P.A.F.H. (ed.) *Sports Injuries: Basic Principles of Prevention and Care*. London: Blackwell Scientific, pp. 417–428.

Denoth, J. (1986) 'Load on the locomotor system and modeling', in Nigg, B.M. (ed.) *Biomechanics of Running Shoes*. Champaign, IL: Human Kinetics, pp. 63–116.

De Wit, B., De Clercq, D. and Aerts, P. (2000) 'Biomechanical analysis of the stance phase during barefoot and shod running', *Journal of Biomechanics*, 33: 269–278.

Dixon, S. J. and Cooke, A. (2004) 'Shoe–surface interaction in tennis', in Hung, G. K. and Pallis, J. M. (eds), *Biomedical Engineering Principles in Sports*. New York: Kluwer Academic/Penum Publishers.

Dixon, S. J. and Stiles, V. H. (2003) 'Impact absorption of tennis shoe–surface combinations', *Sports Engineering*, 6: 1–10.

Dixon, S. J., Batt, M. E. and Collop, A. C. (1999) 'Artificial playing surfaces research: A review of medical, engineering and biomechanical aspects', *International Journal of Sports Medicine*, 20: 209–218.

Dixon, S. J., Collop, A. C. and Batt, M. E. (2000) 'Surface effects on ground reaction forces and lower extremity kinematics in running', *Medicine and Science in Sports and Exercise*, 32: 1919–1926.

Dixon, S. J., James, I. T., Blackburn, K., Pettican, N. and Low, D. (2008) 'Influence of footwear and soil density on loading within the shoe and soil surface during running', *Proceedings of the Institution of Mechanical Engineers, Part P: Journal of Sports Engineering and Technology*, 222: 1–10.

Dura, J. V., Hoyos, J. V., Martinez, A. and Lozano, L. (1999) 'The influence of friction on sports surfaces and turning movements', *Sports Engineering*, 2: 97–102.

Easterling, K. E. (1993) *Advanced Materials for Sports Equipment*. London: Chapman and Hall.

Elvin, N. G., Elvin, A. A., Arnoczky, S. P. and Torry, M. R. (2007) 'The correlation of segment accelerations and impact forces with knee angle in jump landing', *Journal of Applied Biomechanics*, 23: 203–212.

Farley, C. T., Houdijk, H. H., Van Strien, C. and Louie, M. (1998) 'Mechanism of leg stiffness adjustment for hopping on surfaces of different stiffnesses', *Journal of Applied Physiology*, 85: 1044–1055.

Farley, C. T. and Morgenroth, D. C. (1999) 'Leg stiffness primarily depends on ankle stiffness during human hopping', *Journal of Biomechanics*, 32: 267–273.

Feehery, R.V.J. (1986) 'The biomechanics of running on different surfaces', *Clinics in Podiatric Medicine and Surgery*, 3: 649–659.

Ferris, D. P., Louie, M. and Farley, C. T. (1998) 'Running in the real world: Adjusting leg stiffness for different surfaces', *Proceedings of the Royal Society B: Biological Sciences*, 265: 989–994.

Ferris, D.P., Liang, K. & Farley, C.T. (1999) 'Runners adjust leg stiffness for their first step on a new running surface', *Journal of Biomechanics*, 32: 787–794.

Gollhofer, A. (1987) 'Innervation characteristics of m. gastrocnemius during landing on different surfaces', in Jonsson, B. (ed.) *Biomechanics X-B*. Champaign, IL: Human Kinetics, pp. 701–706.

Hagen, M., Homme, A. K., Umlauf, T. and Hennig, E. M. (2010) 'Effects of different shoe-lacing patterns on dorsal pressure distribution during running and perceived comfort', *Research in Sports Medicine*, 18: 176–187.

Hamill, J. and Knutzen, K. M. (2008) *Biomechanial Basis of Human Movement*. Philadelphia, PA: Lippincott Williams & Wilkins.

Hardin, E. C., van den Bogert, A. J. and Hamill, J. (2004) 'Kinematic adaptations during running: Effects of footwear, surface, and duration', *Medicine and Science in Sports and Exercise*, 36: 838–844.

Hennig, E. and Sterzing, T. (2010) 'The influence of soccer shoe design on playing performance: A series of biomechanical studies', *Footwear Science*, 2: 3–11.

Herzog, W. and Leonard, T. R. (1991) 'Validation of optimization models that estimate the forces exerted by synergistic muscles', *Journal of Biomechanics*, 24 (Suppl 1): 31–39.

Hobara, H., Muraoka, T., Omuro, K., Gomi, K. and Sakamoto, M. *et al.* (2009) 'Knee stiffness is a major determinant of leg stiffness during maximal hopping', *Journal of Biomechanics*, 42: 1768–1771.

Hof, A. L. (1992) 'An explicit expression for the moment in multibody systems', *Journal of Biomechanics*, 25: 1209–1211.

Indesteege, J., Camargo, R. E., Mackey, P. W., Bagaglio, G. and Dent, A. (1998) 'Considerations on the selection of polyurethane systems for midsole wedges in athletic footwear application', *Journal of Cellular Plastics,* 34: 329–348.

James, D. I. (1980) 'A broader look at pedestrian friction', *Rubber Chemistry and Technology*, 53: 512–541.

Kälin, X., Denoth, J., Stacoff, A. and Stüssi, E. (1985) 'Cushioning during running', in Perren, S. M. and Schneider, E. (eds), *Biomechanics: Current Interdisciplinary Research*. Dordrecht: Martinus Nijhoff, pp. 651–656.

Kälin, X., Stacoff, A. and Stüssi, E. (1989) 'Torsion and rearfoot stability in running', *Journal of Biomechanics*, 22: 1032.

Kugler, F. and Janshen, L. (2010) 'Body position determines propulsive forces in accelerated running', *Journal of Biomechanics*, 43: 343–348.

Kwon, Y. H. (2008) 'Measurement for deriving kinematic parameters: Numerical methods', in Hong, Y. and Bartlett, R. (eds) *Handbook of Biomechanics and Human Movement Science*. Abingdon: Routledge, pp. 156–181.

Lafortune, M. A., Hennig, E. M. and Lake, M. J. (1996) 'Dominant role of interface over knee angle for cushioning impact loading and regulating initial leg stiffness', *Journal of Biomechanics*, 29: 1523–1529.

Luethi, S. M. and Stacoff, A. (1987) 'The influence of the shoe on foot mechanics in running', in Van Gheluwe, B. and Atha, J. (eds) *Current Research in Sports Biomechanics*. Basel: Karger, pp. 70–85.

Luethi, S. M., Denoth, J., Kälin, X., Stacoff, A. and Stuessi, L. (1987) 'The influence of the shoe on foot movement and shock attenuation in running', in Jonsson, B. (ed.) *Biomechanics X*. Champaign, IL: Human Kinetics.

Luo, G. and Stefanyshyn, D. (2011a) 'Mechanically available traction as a limiting factor to curve sprinting performance', *Footwear Science*, 3: S100–S101.

Luo, G. and Stefanyshyn, D. (2011b) 'Identification of critical traction values for maximum athletic performance', *Footwear Science*, 3: 127–138.

Ly, Q. H., Alaoui, A., Erlicher, S. and Baly, L. (2010) 'Towards a footwear design tool: Influence of shoe midsole properties and ground stiffness on the impact force during running', *Journal of Biomechanics*, 43: 310–317.

McMahon, T. A. and Cheng, G. C. (1990) 'The mechanics of running: How does stiffness couple with speed?', *Journal of Biomechanics*, 23, Suppl 1: 65–78.

McMahon, T. A., Valiant, G. and Frederick, E. C. (1987) 'Groucho running', *Journal of Applied Physiology*, 62: 2326–2337.

McNitt-Gray, J. L., Yokoi, T. and Millward, C. (1993) 'Landing strategy adjustments made by female gymnasts in response to drop height and mat composition', *Journal of Applied Biomechanics*, 9: 173–190.

McNitt-Gray, J. L., Yokoi, T. and Millward, C. (1994) 'Landing strategies used by gymnasts on different surfaces', *Journal of Applied Biomechanics*, 10: 237–252.

McPoil, T. G. (2000) 'Athletic footwear: Design, performance and selection issues', *Journal of Science and Medicine in Sport*, 3: 260–267.

Michel, F. I., Kälin, X.A.M., Westphal, K., Schweizer, F., Campe, S. and Segesser, B. (2009) 'The functional sport shoe parameter "torsion" within running shoe research – a literature review', *Sportverletzung, Sportschaden*, 23: 9.

Mills, N. J. (2007) Chapter 13 – Running shoe case study', in *Polymer Foams Handbook: Engineering and Biomechanics Applications and Design Guide*. Oxford: Butterworth-Heinemann, pp. 307–327.

Morin, J. B., Edouard, P. and Samozino, P. (2011) 'Technical ability of force application as a determinant factor of sprint performance', *Medicine and Science in Sports and Exercise*, 43: 1680–1688.

Morio, C., Lake, M. J., Gueguen, N., Rao, G. and Baly, L. (2009) 'The influence of footwear on foot motion during walking and running', *Journal of Biomechanics*, 42: 2081–2088.

Moritz, C. T. and Farley, C. T. (2004) 'Passive dynamics change leg mechanics for an unexpected surface during human hopping', *Journal of Applied Physiology*, 97: 1313–1322.

Nigg, B. M. (1983) 'External force measurements with sport shoes and playing surfaces', in Nigg, B. M. and Kerr, B. A. (eds), *International Symposium on Biomechanical Aspects of Sport Shoes and Playing Surfaces*. Calgary: University Printing, pp. 11–24.

Nigg, B. M. (2010) 'Impact force, soft-tissue vibrations, and muscle tuning'. In *Biomechanics of Sports Shoes*. Calgary: University of Calgary , pp. 47–78.

Nigg, B. M. and Liu, W. (1999) 'The effect of muscle stiffness and damping on simulated impact force peaks during running', *Journal of Biomechanics*, 32: 849–856.

Nigg, B. M. and Morlock, M. (1987) 'The influence of lateral heel flare of running shoes on pronation and impact forces', *Medicine and Science in Sports and Exercise*, 19: 294–302.

Nigg, B. M. and Yeadon, M. R. (1987) 'Biomechanical aspects of playing surfaces', *Journal of Sports Science*, 5: 117–145.

Nigg, B., Bahlsen, A., Denoth, J., Luethi, S. M. and Stacoff, A. (1986) 'Factors influencing kinetic and kinematic variables in running', in Nigg, B. M. (ed.), *Biomechanics of Running Shoes*. Champaign, IL: Human Kinetics Publishers, pp. 139–159.

Nigg, B. M., Bahlsen, H. A., Luethi, S. M. and Stokes, S. (1987) 'The influence of running velocity and midsole hardness on external impact forces in heel-toe running', *Journal of Biomechanics*, 20: 951–959.

Nigg, B. M., Cole, G. K. and Bruggemann, G. P. (1995) 'Impact forces during heel toe running', *Journal of Applied Biomechanics*, 11: 407–432.

Nigg, B. M., Stefanyshyn, D. J., Rozitis, A. I. and Mündermann, A. (2009) 'Resultant knee joint moments for lateral movement tasks on sliding and non-sliding sport surfaces', *Journal of Sports Science*, 27, 427–435.

Nikooyan, A. A. and Zadpoor, A. A. (2011) 'Mass-spring-damper modelling of the human body to study running and hopping – an overview', *Proceedings of the Institution of Mechanical Engineers, Part H: Journal of Engineering in Medicine*, 225: 1121–1135.

Nilsson, J., Thorstensson, A. and Halbertsma, J. (1985) 'Changes in leg movements and muscle activity with speed of locomotion and mode of progression in humans', *Acta Physiologica Scandinavica*, 123: 457–475.

Perry, S. D. and Lafortune, M. A. (1995) 'Influences of inversion/eversion of the foot upon impact loading during locomotion', *Clinical Biomechanics*, 10: 253–257.

Sanders, R. H. and Allen, J. B. (1993) 'Changes in net joint torques during accomodation to change in surface compliance in a drop jumping task', *Human Movement Science*, 12: 299–326.

Shiba, N., Kitaoka, H. B., Cahalan, T. D. and Chao, E. Y. (1995) 'Shock-absorbing effect of shoe insert materials commonly used in management of lower extremity disorders', *Clinical Orthopaedics and Related Research*, 130–136.

Shorten, M. R. (1993) 'The energetics of running and running shoes', *Journal of Biomechanics*, 26, Suppl 1: 41–51.

Shorten, M. R. (2002) 'The myth of running shoe cushioning', 4th International Conference of Engineering of Sport, Kyoto, Japan, 3–6 September 2002.

Shorten, M. and Mientjes, M. (2011) 'The "heel impact" force peak during running is neither "heel" nor "impact" and does not quantify shoe cushioning effects', *Footwear Science*, 3: 41–58.

Squadrone, R. and Gallozzi, C. (2009) 'Biomechanical and physiological comparison of barefoot and two shod conditions in experienced barefoot runners', *Journal of Sports Medicine and Physical Fitness*, 49: 6–13.

Stacoff, A., Kälin, X., Stüssi, E. and Segesser, B. (1989) 'The torsion of the foot in running', *International Journal of Sport Biomechanics*, 5: 375–389.

Stacoff, A., Kalin, X. and Stussi, E. (1991) 'The effects of shoes on the torsion and rearfoot motion in running', *Medicine and Science in Sports and Exercise*, 23: 482–490.

Sterzing, T., Muller, C., Hennig, E. and Milani, T. (2009) 'Actual and perceived running performance in soccer shoes: A series of eight studies', *Footwear Science*, 1: 5–17.

Sterzing, T., Muller, C. and Milani, T. (2010) 'Traction on artificial turf: Development of a soccer shoe outsole', *Footwear Science*, 2: 37–49.

Stucke, H., Baudzu, W. and Baumann, W. (1984) 'On friction characteristics of playing surfaces', in Frederick, E. C. (ed.) *Sport Shoes and Playing Surfaces: Biomechanical Properties*. Champaign, IL: Human Kinetics, pp. 87–97.

Tessutti, V., Trombini-Souza, F., Ribeiro, A. P., Nunes, A. L. and Sacco Ide, C. (2010) 'In-shoe plantar pressure distribution during running on natural grass and asphalt in recreational runners', *Journal of Science and Medicine in Sport*, 13: 151–155.

Thompson, C. and Raibert, M. (1990) 'Passive dynamic running', in Hayward, V. and Khatib, O. (eds) *Experimental Robotics I*, vol. 139. Berlin/Heidelberg; Cambridge, MA: Springer, pp. 74–83.

Valiant, G. A. (1987) 'The relationship between normal pressure and the friction developed by shoe outsole material on a court surface', *Journal of Biomechanics*, 20: 892.

Valiant, G. (1990) 'Traction characteristics of outsoles for use on artificial playing surfaces', in Schmidt, R. C., Hoerner, E. F., Milner, E. M. and Morehouse, C. A. (eds), *Natural and Artificial Playing Fields: Characteristics and Safety Features*. Philadelphia: American Society for Testing and Materials, pp. 61–68.

Van Gheluwe, B., Kerwin, D., Roosen, P. and Tielemans, R. (1999) 'The influence of heel fit on rearfoot motion in running shoes', *Journal of Applied Biomechanics*, 15: 361–372.

Weyand, P. G., Sternlight, D. B., Bellizzi, M. J. and Wright, S. (2000) 'Faster top running speeds are achieved with greater ground forces not more rapid leg movements', *Journal of Applied Physiology*, 89: 1991–1999.

Wilson, J. F., Rochelle, R. D. and Bischoff, J. E. (1997) 'Identification and correlation of human footfall load parameters using multivariate analysis', *Journal of Biomechanical Engineering*, 119: 115–123.

Windle, C. M., Gregory, S. M. and Dixon, S. J. (1999) 'The shock attenuation characteristics of four different insoles when worn in a military boot during running and marching', *Gait Posture*, 9: 31–37.

Wright, I. C., Neptune, R. R., van den Bogert, A. J. and Nigg, B. M. (1997) 'Passive regulation of impact forces in heel-toe running', 3rd Symposium on Footwear Biomechanics, Tokyo, August 1997.

Young, C. and Fleming, P. R. (2007) 'A review of mechanical impact testing devices for sport surfaces'. Paper presented at the international conference 'Sport Technology and Research into Sport Surfaces – STARSS', CD-ROM, Loughborough University, September 2007, editors Fleming, P. R., Carre, M. J., Dixon, S. J. and James, I. Available at: http://sportsurf.lboro.ac.uk

Chapter 8

# Natural turf sports surfaces

*Iain James*

## Introduction

Natural turf has, for a long time, been *the* surface for outdoor sport. This is changing with the development of synthetic turf surfaces, most notably in field hockey but increasingly in football and even rugby. Natural turf surfaces continue to develop however. Consider the natural turf surfaces of 30 years ago, surfaces that would turn from autumn splendour to winter quagmire with very little rainfall, and require players to change shirts at half time so they could be identified. Such occurrences are rare in modern elite-level sport, but persist at the recreational level. Advances have been made in the construction and drainage of natural turf surfaces and more recently in the management of the growing environment for the turf plant. It is important to remember that the performance of sports surfaces is not just a question of the mechanics of the constituent materials but also of the biological performance of the turf plant itself.

Natural turf remains the benchmark for performance and safety for many sports such as football and rugby. The biggest limitation of natural turf, however, is that it has a low resistance to wear, resulting in a low sustainable carrying capacity (hours of use per week without irrecoverable detriment to surface quality). This is because the turf plant is a living organism that requires the right quantity and quality of structural support, light, air and water to be resilient to the stresses applied in use. These requirements are commonly compromised, leading to reduced wear resistance. Increasing the carrying capacity of natural turf surfaces at all levels of sport is the focus for engineers and scientists working in the continued development of these surfaces. A natural turf surface is a complex system integrating the plant with a granular soil rootzone that varies in space and time in response to environmental variables. This chapter considers the complexity of this system and how it can be optimised for improved surface performance.

## The turfgrass plant

The requirements of turf grasses are common to those of most plants: light, water, $CO_2$, $O_2$, nutrients and structural support in a rootzone (Figure 8.1). Above ground, the leaves of the grass intercept light of between 400 and 700nm and carbon dioxide for photosynthesis; oxygen and water vapour are emitted through the leaf structure. This gas and water exchange is reversed below ground where respiration in the root system consumes $O_2$ and emits $CO_2$. Respiration also takes place through the leaf structure in the absence of light. Water movement into the roots and up through the plant is driven by transpiration, a plant controlled process that creates a potential through the plant structure for water to move from the soil into the roots, through the plant and out through

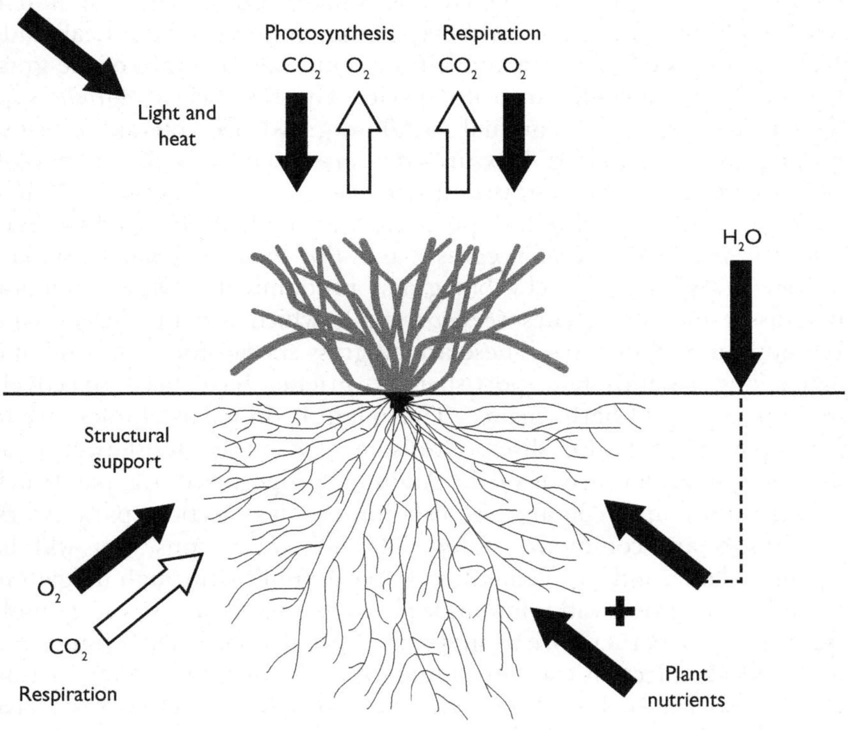


*Figure 8.1* A simplified diagram of the essential requirements of the turfgrass plant, which include solar light and heat, above-ground exchange of $CO_2$ and $O_2$, sufficient water from precipitation and/or irrigation to infiltrate into the soil rootzone and be drawn into the plant through its root system, along with essential plant nutrients. There must also be sufficient air-filled porosity to allow respiration within the rootzone.

the leaves. This transpiring water provides rigidity to the plant from cellular turgor pressure. Nutrients are drawn into the root structure from the soil by osmosis and transported along with other biochemicals such as hormones to other cells around the plant.

The natural growth and development cycle for a grass species is from seed germination, to establishment, to the production of a seed head and in the case of annuals, mortality, or in perennials, dormancy and further reproduction. This typical growth cycle is interrupted in the management of sports turf by routine, frequent mowing of the grass. Grass mowing heights reflect the type of sport being played. On surfaces where ball roll is critical, such as golf greens or lawn bowling greens, the grass will be mown closely (3–mm in height). Mowing height increases as ball roll becomes less critical and wear resistance and impact reduction become the principal requirements, such that mowing height will be 20–35mm in football, 35–50mm in rugby and over 75mm in horse racing. Leaf blade characteristics such as width and stiffness, and the tolerance of the grass plant to close mowing, vary with species. Grasses such as *Agrostis* spp. (bents) and *Poa annua* (annual meadow grass) are tolerant to close mowing and have fine leaf textures that are suitable for fast-paced ball roll on golf greens. Such grasses are lower in wear tolerance and divot easily so are less suitable for sports such as football and rugby where *Loleum perenne* (perennial ryegrass) and *Poa pratensis* (smooth-stalked meadow grass or Kentucky bluegrass) predominate. Other common turfgrasses include fescues (*Festuca* spp.), which are fine-leaved and common on golf fairways. These are all grass species found in wild and managed grasslands but sport-specific varieties have been selectively bred for improved performance. This might be in terms of tolerance to close mowing but also disease resistance, drought resistance, wear resistance and tolerance of shade. Aesthetic properties of the plant such as leaf width and colour are also important selection parameters. Turfgrasses are commonly water deficient for reasons that will be explained later, and supplementary water is applied through irrigation. Reducing water demand is important because quality water is commonly a scarce resource, therefore drought tolerance is a particularly important trait. Species selection can also influence water demand. Warm-season ($C_4$) grass species such as *Cynodon dactylon* (couch or Bermuda grass) have a modified photosynthetic pathway that is different from cool season ($C_3$) grasses such as those named above. As a consequence they are more heat and drought tolerant but become dormant at lower temperatures at which cool season grasses are still actively growing. Therefore they are only suitable for certain climates or certain times of the year (summer periods). In transitional zones between warm and cool season grass climates, warm season grasses are commonly over-sown with cool season grasses in the winter.

During play the grass must be resilient to the compressive and shear stresses applied by participants and to ball impacts and shear stresses from equipment such as sticks used in Gaelic sports and occasionally field hockey (although this a sport almost exclusively played on short-pile synthetic turf surfaces due to ball roll characteristics and resilience to stick strike). A healthy plant with a deep and extensive root system is more able to resist these stresses because a greater volume of soil is exploited for water and nutrients, and the anchorage of the plant is increased. The maintenance of natural turf is not simply the production of the correct grass leaf height through mowing; the natural turf surface manager must also ensure that there is sufficient water, nutrients and oxygen for the plant root system and sufficient light and $CO_2$ above ground for photosynthesis. Because this is an organic system that is prevented from reproduction, seeding or turf replacement is necessary to replace worn turf with desirable species. Weed plants and grass species compete for water and nutrient resources and have an adverse impact on performance and aesthetics so are typically controlled with herbicides and cultural practices. Stressed plants are susceptible to disease from fungal pathogens so turf maintenance also includes prophylactic and reactive fungicide application. This can result in environmental load from maintenance and is increasingly unpopular with surface users.

Reduction of photosynthetically active radiation from the sun is common due to shading problems from trees and buildings. At the recreational level this is less common but has to be considered in the design of golf courses, where trees form both landscape feature and hazard, and most acutely in the design of stadia for elite-level sport. In evolutionary terms, grasses have been one of the most successful plants, being able to colonise a range of environments but the high-usage stadium environment remains a significant challenge. High-sided, large-capacity stadia shade the pitch from the sun and at high latitudes this can be a problem that leads to the pitch receiving less than an hour of direct sunlight in winter months, usually when usage is greatest. Stadium design has been modified to address this. Where space and capital permit, the pitch can be constructed on a removable tray that can slide out to a less shaded side of the stadium to receive more sunlight to aid recovery. A less expensive and arguably less effective method is to include panelling in roofing structures that transmit light in the 400–700nm waveband. An increasingly popular method is to use growth lighting, adapted from glasshouse technology, to provide intensive supplementary light to the pitch. Lighting rigs, with bulbs emitting light in the correct frequency range, are attached to wheeled aluminium rigs that cover around 350 $m^2$ each and are moved around the pitch when not in use to reduce the impact of shade. This improves grass health and recovery from wear but increases energy consumption.

## The soil system

The role of the soil system in supporting turfgrass function has already been introduced when considering the requirements of the plant. It is essential for the plant to provide oxygen, water and nutrients to the plant root system, which must also be able to develop into the soil to gain structural support and anchorage. The soil also performs mechanical functions in terms of the player–surface interaction and ball–surface interaction that will be explored later.

Soils used in natural turf sports surfaces comprise a granular mineral skeleton that can be characterised by its particle-size distribution within three principal size fractions: sand 2mm to 63$\mu$m and typically silica or calcite; silt 63$\mu$m to 2$\mu$m, a combination of mechanically weathered silica and phyllosilicates; and clay $<2\mu$m, typically phyllosilicates. The sand fraction can be determined by wet sieving and is commonly divided into 3–5 sub fractions. The silt and clay fractions are determined from their settling times in water as described by Stoke's law (see ISO 11277 (2009) for further details). Soils are commonly classified according to the relative proportions of these three major particle-size fractions (Figure 8.2; James, 2011). The relative proportions, arrangement and mineralogy of these particle-size fractions have a significant effect on the physical and mechanical behaviour of the soil, which ultimately determines pitch performance. There is also an organic fraction of the soil formed from living soil microbiology and dead and decaying plant and animal matter. The organic matter content of soil can be determined by mass balance following combustion at 450°C. The organic matter fraction provides nutrients to the plant and retains water and nutrients in the soil.

Packing of mineral and organic particles in a soil results in the formation of a pore network within the granular bulk soil. It follows that this pore network has a size distribution and connectivity that is a function of the particle-size distribution and the packing density of the particles. Following rainfall, water will infiltrate into the pore network of a soil under gravity and a tension created by capillary action as water is attracted to the dry surface of the pore. Infiltrating water displaces gas within the soil. When all the pores are filled with water, the soil is termed *saturated* and is anoxic, i.e. there is no oxygen for plant root or soil microbe respiration and the turf plant becomes stressed. Typically the water content of a soil is in flux in response to climatic variables including precipitation and temperature due to evapotranspiration (the combined effects of evaporation and plant transpiration). Soil water movement is determined by hydraulic potential within the soil, a balance of gravitational potential and a pore potential that is either negative in unsaturated pores or positive when the soil is saturated and pressure heads build up. Typically, the larger the pore space, the more easily water moves

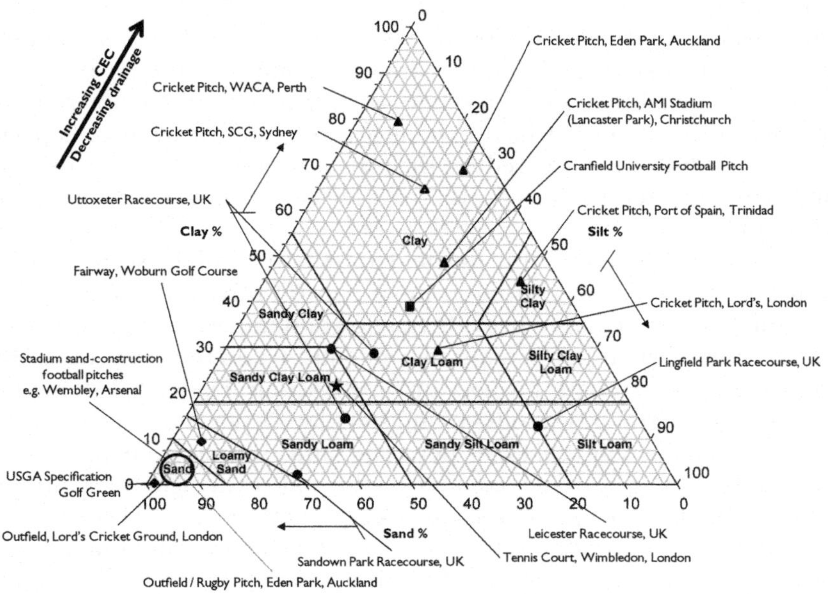


*Figure 8.2* The classification of soils commonly used in sports surfaces by the proportion of sand (2mm–63μm), silt (63μm–2μm) and clay (<2μm) particle sizes, CEC is the cation exchange capacity of the soil. Reproduced from James, I. T., *Proceedings of the Institution of Mechanical Engineers Part P: J. Sports Engineering and Technology*, 225, pp. 115–129, © 2011 Sage Publishing. Reprinted by permission of SAGE.

downwards due to gravitational potential and the greater the rate of water movement. Water flow rates within the soil are proportional to the hydraulic conductivity of a soil, a rate constant that is a function of pore size (and therefore particle size and packing), pore connectivity and the degree of saturation. Thus soils with a large proportion of sand particles (Figure 8.2) are more freely draining and have greater infiltration rates than soils with a large proportion of clay particles. This is advantageous in that it is easier to maintain aerobic conditions within the soil but has two drawbacks in that it is difficult to retain sufficient water for plant turgor and health, and soluble nutrients are easily removed through drainage water from the soil (a process known as leaching).

To reduce leaching it is necessary to either reduce drainage from the soil or decrease the solubility of nutrients into the soil solution. Cation exchange capacity is a property of a soil that describes its capacity to exchange plant-essential nutrient cations with the soil solution. The cations are held by electrostatic attraction to the surface of certain clay minerals, which due to their mineralogical structure and weathering have a negative surface charge, and also in complexes with organic matter. The cation exchange capacity of a sand soil is extremely low and as a consequence sand soils have low nutrient status. Amendment of sand soils with organic matter is a common strategy to improve the fertility of the soils but inevitably higher quantities of nutrient fertiliser are required compared to clay soils which exhibit greater cation exchange capacity. Coated fertiliser products reduce the rate at which the fertiliser dissolves into solution, reducing the risk of nutrient supply exceeding plant demand.

So in terms of water and nutrient retention it might seem that clay would be the ideal soil selection for a natural turf sports surface. The natural turf surface has to provide traction and impact energy absorption for the player when performing movements. To do this it needs to have sufficient shear strength for boot or shoe traction. Figure 8.3 shows how the shear strength of two soils, a sand soil (98:1:1 per cent sand: silt: clay) and a clay loam soil (29:45:26 per cent sand: silt: clay) changes as the saturation ratio (the water content of the soil divided by its saturation water content) increases. The shear strength of the sand soil remains high over a range of saturation ratio from 0.3 to 0.8. The shear strength of the clay is lower and decreases rapidly with increasing water content. This is the essential difference between sand and clay soils – their shear strength

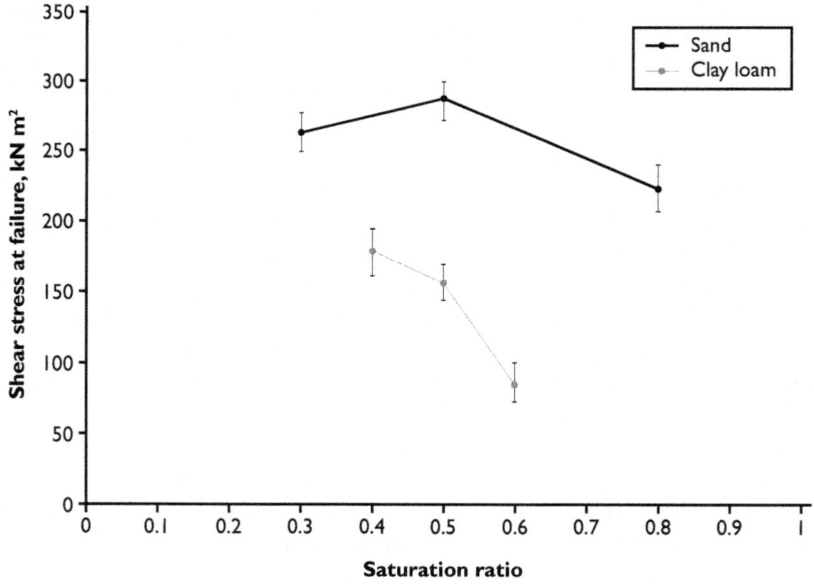


*Figure 8.3* Shear stress at failure with increasing saturation ratio in triaxial testing of two soils used in sports surfaces at 100kPa confining stress. Based on data from Guisasola *et al.* (2010a).

and the sensitivity of that shear strength to water content. While a clay loam provides a better environment for a grass plant in terms of water and nutrient retention, unless it is very dry, as soon as it is loaded it will fail and it will fail plastically resulting in turf detachment (divoting), surface deformation and localised compaction. A sand soil will prove more resilient in most precipitation conditions although irrigation and fertiliser inputs will be required to prevent drought and nutrient stress in the plant. Furthermore the saturation ratio and shear strength of a sand soil are likely to be more spatially consistent because of their resistance to compaction and relatively high infiltration rate and hydraulic conductivity. Rapid transport of water from the surface to drainage at depth means that the water content at the surface is lower after a precipitation event, maintaining shear strength in the contact zone between players and the surface. Where water is allowed to pond, significant plastic deformation of the soil takes place during use, further reducing the infiltration rate, thus a negative cycle of pitch deterioration begins. As a result, for the majority of sports, sand is the preferred rootzone soil material (Figure 8.2).

This is not the case in sports such as cricket and tennis where ball bounce is more important than player traction (Figure 8.2). In these sports, densely packed, dry clay soils are used because they have a high stiffness in this state. Consequently these surfaces can only be used in the summer when precipitation is low and evapotranspiration high, such that water content is low. At very low water contents, the shear strength and stiffness of a clay soil increases significantly. This means that the hardness of the surface increases and plastic deformation on ball impact is reduced significantly, resulting in a greater coefficient of restitution between ball and surface. Hardness increases to such an extent that cricket players wear spiked (2–4mm diameter) rather than studded footwear, and tennis players use dimple-soled rubber shoes to generate traction between the shoe and the grass-soil surface.

So it can be seen that material selection is important in the construction of natural turf surfaces. To describe the performance of a natural turf surface, it is essential to characterise the materials used in its construction. As a minimum this should comprise determination of the particle-size distribution, bulk density (packing), water content and organic matter content. These properties of a surface can vary in three dimensions. In constructed surfaces, spatial variation can be expected to be minimal compared to the majority of natural turf systems which have been levelled and fashioned from agricultural grassland systems and where spatial variation in soil type and properties can be significant, even at a 7000m$^2$ pitch scale. Variation of these properties through the profile should also be considered – a 20mm layer of sand over a 280mm clay profile will behave like a clay, not like a 300mm deep sand profile. It should also be emphasised that to classify a 'natural turf surface' without reference to the sport being played is foolhardy. One of the advantages of natural turf is that the components can be varied to suit a particular sport, whether it is the grass type across the different playing surfaces of a golf course or the contrast between a clay surface for the cricket pitch, where the ball bounces, and a sand surface for the outfield, where ball bounce is less critical than player traction and wear resistance (see also Chapter 2).

## Design and construction

### *Elite and recreational-level natural turf surfaces*

While the majority of focus is on the quality and performance of elite-level natural turf facilities such as football stadia, baseball parks, cricket grounds, championship golf courses or Wimbledon's tennis courts, the majority of natural turf surfaces are not constructed from materials offsite but are simply formed from the native soil and seeded or turfed with turfgrass cultivars of suitable grass species. This has the advantage of reducing material costs and transport, a typical sand football pitch construction of 70m x 100m x 0.4m depth would require 4,480 tonnes of soil material (at a dry density of 1600kg $m^{-3}$) but has the disadvantage that surface behaviour will be determined by the material characteristics and this is commonly to the detriment of surface quality if the native soil has a high clay content.

Constructed profiles typically comprise a sand rootzone overlying a gravel drainage layer, which in turn overlies a drainage pipe network (see Chapter 2). The principle of the design is that in a partially saturated state, water is retained within the sand due to pore capillarity. This creates a suspended water table in the sand, over the gravel, allowing the plant to access water. During a rainfall event a positive water pressure builds over the interface between the sand and gravel and forces water into the freely draining gravel and ultimately into the drainage system, where water is transported to outfall. The relative sizes of the sand and gravel are critical. If the sand is too coarse, it will not retain a sufficient depth of water for the plant; if it is too fine then it will exhibit excessive water retention and could migrate into the gravel layer, providing hydraulic continuity that will remove the suspended water table. Medium sands of similar diameter are used – by keeping the diameter of particles uniform it reduces the risk of compaction.

Due to its high hydraulic conductivity it is not possible to maintain grass health with this construction approach, without an irrigation system. Water is required for plant health but also to maintain surface strength. Look at Figure 8.3 again and note how the shear strength of the sand soil increases marginally from 0.3 to 0.5 per cent saturation. This is due to apparent cohesion caused by pore water under tension increasing the strength of the soil. This effect diminishes with further addition of water as the pore water tension decreases and eventually becomes positive pressure.

The quantity of irrigation required for maintaining a constructed sand pitch depends on climate but is considerable. Where the availability of water or the cost of irrigation infrastructure is unaffordable then a sand construction surface is inappropriate. A more affordable solution is to use a native soil, and if this has a low hydraulic conductivity provide a surface drainage system. A surface drainage system provides a high hydraulic conductivity conduit between the soil surface and a piped drainage system at depth. A traditional agricultural sub-surface drainage system commonly does not cure problems on a sports surface because it is only designed to lower a near-surface water table. In a sports pitch it is essential to transport water from the surface to the drainage outfall as quickly as possible during and following a precipitation event. For low hydraulic conductivity soils, the only way to achieve this is by bypassing the native soil using a system of sand slits of varying dimensions that intersect the sub-surface drains (Ward, 1983; James *et al.*, 2007). Sand slits are typically sand-filled 400mm-deep, 40mm-wide slits cut in the soil across the length or width of the pitch at an inter-slit spacing of 1–2 m although shallower, narrower slits are sometimes used at 100–200mm spacing (see Chapter 2, Figure 2.1). The slit provides a high hydraulic conductivity route for water to move from the surface, where player–surface interaction takes place, to deeper sub-surface drains. For the surface to function, the slits must be connected to the surface, so it is essential to topdress the whole pitch with sand to a depth of 12–20mm and routinely to provide further sand additions to maintain the hydraulic continuity between surface and sand slit. Without this routine maintenance the slits become capped by the shearing of the native soil during play and the sand slit drains become disconnected from the surface and effectively defunct until the continuity is restored. An alternative approach in suitable clay soils is to form a 50mm diameter channel at 400mm depth using a mole plough. This technique is only suitable in stable clay soils but provides a rapid, cheap form of drainage (for further details of this method see James *et al.*, 2007).

Pitch construction method is a trade-off between the costs of installation and operation, and required level and consistency of performance. An example of the relative costs can be seen by considering the English Premier League, one of the wealthiest club leagues in football. The majority of stadium pitches in the league are constructed sand profiles but the proportion of pitches in their training facilities constructed in this manner is much lower. The training pitches, pitches in lower leagues and the majority of recreational football, are drained native soil, or a sand-ameliorated drained native soil. This is because the construction and operating costs of sand profile pitches are so high. The image of the muddy weekend player still exists in sport, it is just not seen as often on television because of the improved quality of stadium pitches – but this does come at a cost.

### *Hybrid surfaces*

The problem with sand surfaces is that they have low cohesion, their strength comes from inter-particle friction caused by interlocking, rather than inter-particle cohesion that is more common in clay soils. This means that while confined and compacted, sands have a high shear strength; when loose and less confined, their strength reduces, leaving them susceptible to damage from divoting. The grass plant has a critical role in binding the sand soil together to maintain it strength. A number of technologies have been developed to increase the stability or strength of sand soils and can be divided into two broad categories: soil stabilisation and synthetic turf fibre 'hybridisation'. Soil stabilisation is commonly achieved by the inclusion of narrow fibres (35mm length, 0.1mm diameter) of polypropylene or a mix of polypropylene and rubber which aims to bind the soil together, mimicking the effect of fine turf roots. This can increase the strength of a soil (Baker, 1997; McNitt and Landschoot, 2005) but also its hardness and stiffness. Synthetic hybrid methods use synthetic turf fibres that are either punched into the natural turf pitch individually (Figure 8.4) or are tufted into a biodegradable backing, which is then filled with soil and turfed or seeded with grass. The synthetic fibres then sit between the surface and mowing height to reduce the wear on the natural turf fibres and provide some vertical reinforcement of the soil profile. The other advantage of this method is that as the natural turf wears, some green colour remains in the surface.

## Defining and characterising performance

### *Subjective and objective measurement in natural turf*

Chapter 3 shows that for synthetic turf surfaces, the development has been led by sport-specific performance standards that actually aim to match the performance of high-quality natural turf, yet there are limited comparable performance standards for natural turf. Perhaps because it is seen as the benchmark surface and that it has been used for the majority of modern sports since their inception, it is actually rare to find a prescribed performance standard for a natural turf surface, although they are becoming more common. Generally decisions on playability are left to the match officials who use criteria such as 'Can the players move without excessive slipping?' and 'Does the ball roll a reasonable distance?' to determine that a pitch is suitable for play. This is not the case in horse

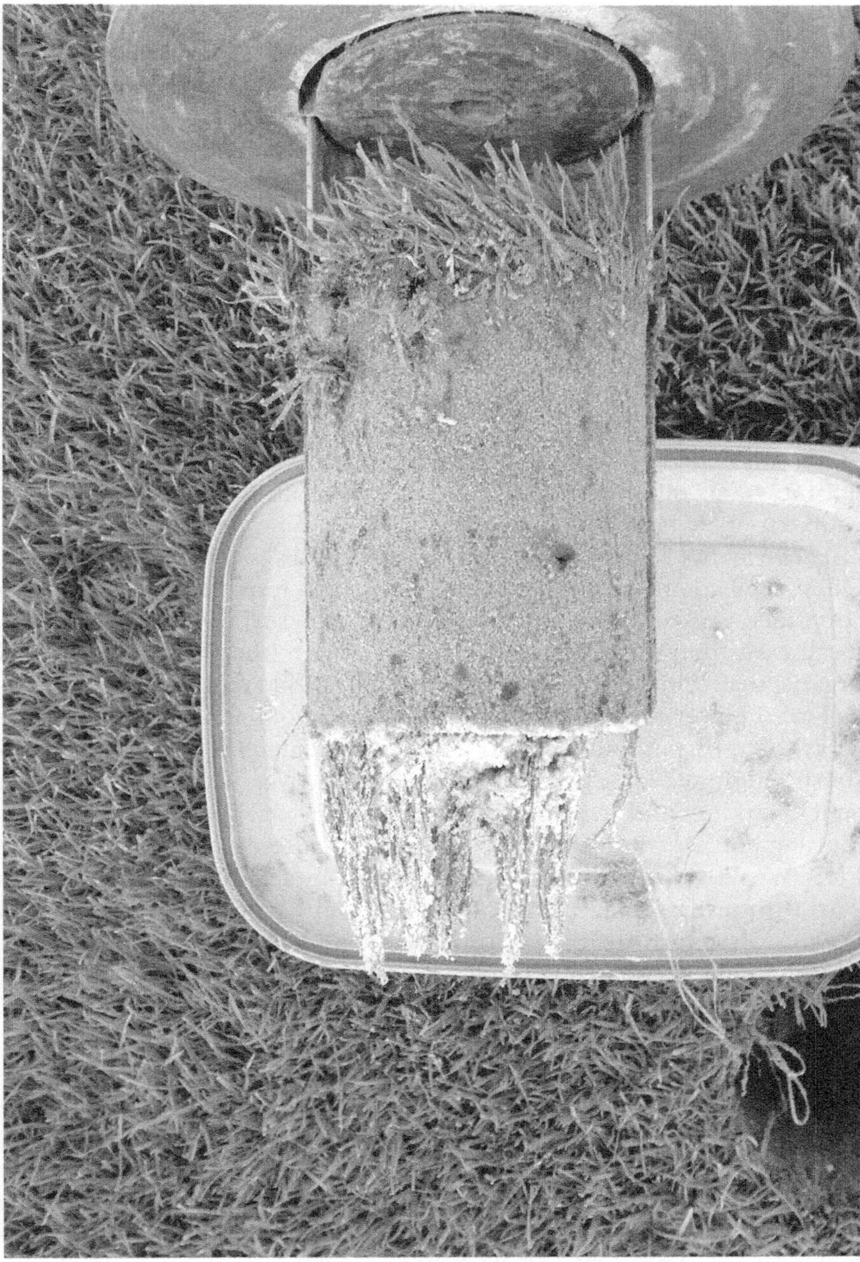

*Figure 8.4* Photograph of a core sample taken from a hybrid Desso Grassmaster pitch. The synthetic turf fibres can be seen to be penetrating through the soil and helping to stabilise the pitch. The grass at the surface is then a mixture of natural and synthetic turf fibres. © TGMS Ltd, 2014.

racing in the UK where limits for surface 'going' are provided by the governing body/regulator, the British Horseracing Authority, which is aiming to reduce the risk of horse injury and race meeting cancellation. Racecourses are obliged to use the GoingStick (Dufour and Mumford, 2008), which measures penetration resistance and shearing resistance of a 100mm x 20mm x 6mm blade inserted into the turf. This objective measurement is used to 'declare' the performance of the racecourse, information that is used by horse trainers, jockeys and spectators to manage horse performance. This is a rare example of objective measurement tools being used in the decision of when a natural turf surface is suitable for sport. Other examples include the use of the 2.25kg Clegg Impact Surface Tester device in Australian rules football, where impact decelerations 120 gravities or over are considered too high (Chivers and Aldous, 2004) leading to ground closures, although a study by Twomey (2010) showed that although there was a relationship between hardness and injury in Australian rules football, it was not necessarily with extremely hard or soft conditions.

Performance standards for natural turf do exist (Sport England, 2011). Often they comprise a large suite of different tests that consider grass coverage, grass colour, incidence of weeds, surface levels, traction, hardness, infiltration rate and thatch content (thatch is accumulated organic matter near the surface of the soil profile that adversely affects ball– and player–surface interactions). It is not common to use such large arrays of testing in routine natural turf management as they are too time-consuming and many of them are subjective. They are used in benchmarking and ensuring standardisation of pitch quality across tournaments, as conducted by the Sports Turf Research Institute for the FIFA World Cup in South Africa 2010 and by the New Zealand Sports Turf Institute in preparation for the 2011 Rugby World Cup. Commercial systems also measure these properties at individual elite venues as a measurement and benchmarking tool throughout the season.

## *Current test methods*

For sports using a relatively large ball that is passed or carried, testing can be reduced to three simple questions: a) Is the surface too hard or too soft?; b) Is there sufficient but not excessive traction; and c) Is the ball–surface interaction suitable? Of course this varies from sport to sport. Football has particular concern regarding traction and ball–surface interaction; golf and cricket are predominantly concerned with ball–surface interaction and hardness. Additional testing might be required to explain variation in these parameters or the cause of unacceptable limits but the development of testing devices should aim to enable routine, objective measurement of these parameters. It needs to recognise that appropriate technology is not necessarily the most complicated but that it needs to be objective, be reliable, allow rapid measurement and be affordable.

Two commonly used devices are the Clegg Impact Surface Tester and the studded-plate traction device (see also Chapter 3). The Clegg Impact Surface Tester comprises a uniaxial accelerometer within a cylindrical aluminium missile that is dropped from a fixed height and the peak deceleration on impact determined. The mass and drop height of the missile vary but the most common configuration is a 2.25kg hammer dropped from 450mm (alternatives include 0.5kg from 550mm and 4.5kg from 450mm). Recommended suitable hardnesses vary from sport to sport, as discussed above. The studded-plate testing device has been in use in sports surface testing since the 1980s (Canaway and Bell, 1986). The device is a modification of the bevameter used in terramechanics to determine the trafficability of soils and comprises a steel disc with a uniform stud pattern that is loaded with 46 ± 2kg dropped from 60 ± 5mm and then rotated at a constant speed manually and the peak torque recorded (BS EN 15301-1, 2007). Adaptations of this device log torque with angle of rotation but the majority of 'standards' provide ranges for peak torque. While this device is relatively simple to manufacture it has the drawback of having a total mass of approximately 55kg, limiting portability in manual operation. Alternative approaches to measuring traction include using a simple shear vane or devices that measure a shearing resistance such as the GoingStick, although these devices cannot determine the effect of variation in stud type and stud pattern.

Properties such as hardness and traction should be expected to change over time on natural turf surfaces because of the way the organic plant, and both organic and inorganic soil materials, respond to variations in wear, compaction and weather. This was illustrated in work published by Caple *et al.* (2012) which showed how surface construction and maintenance resulted in different degrees of spatial and temporal variation. Figure 8.5 shows how sand construction elite-level natural turf surfaces have greater hardness than natural soil surfaces, but that this property is more consistent in space and time in the elite surface. Figure 8.6 shows that there is a change in shear resistance when the sand construction pitch (C) becomes drier, but that it is more spatially uniform.

Quantifying the suitability of ball–surface interaction is more complex and varies from sport to sport (see also Chapter 3). Ball roll behaviour can be determined by rolling a ball down a standard ramp and measuring the distance the ball travels before coming to rest, additionally the deviation of the ball from a straight trajectory may also be recorded and more sophisticated devices can measure ball deceleration over a 1–2m distance from the base of the ramp. Standards set minimum and maximum limits for ball roll distance, based on the assumption that given a standard

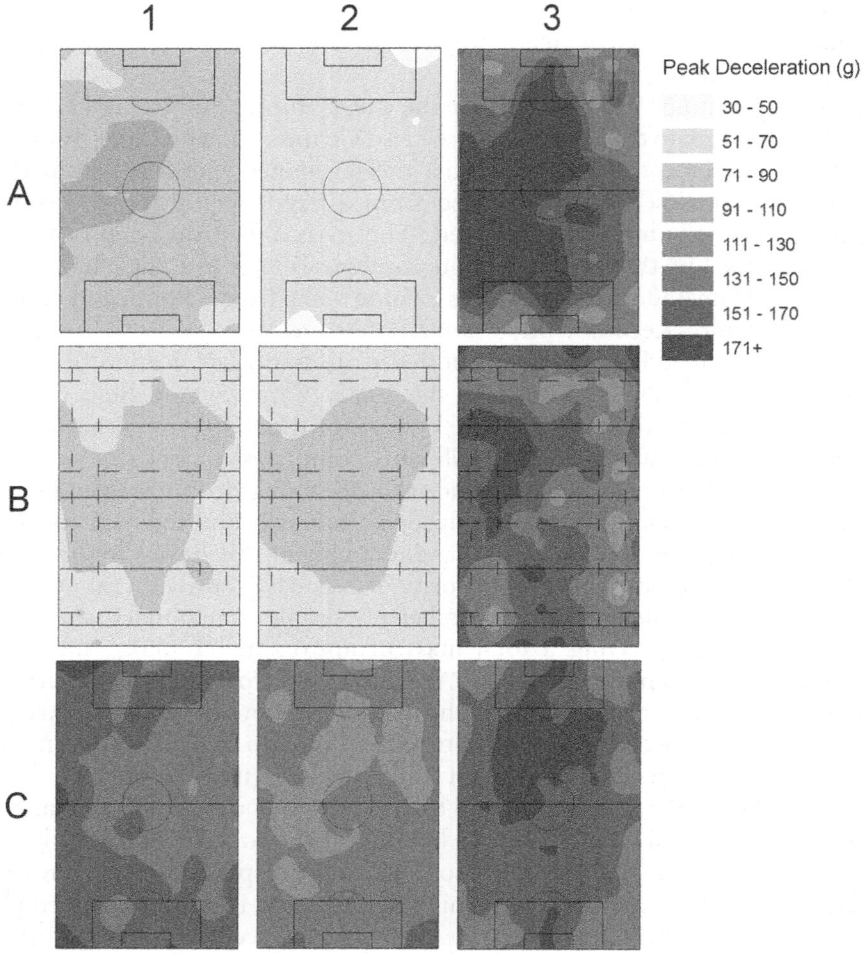


*Figure 8.5* Maps of peak deceleration measured with the Clegg Impact Surface Tester from the three pitches (A: recreational-level association football, natural clay soil; B: tier 2 professional rugby, sand dressed clay soil; and C: tier 2 professional association football, sand construction hybrid surface) at three times across the season (1 = beginning of season – September; 2 = mid-season –January; 3 = end of season – April/May). Reproduced from Caple et al. (2012), © International Sports Engineering Association, with kind permission of Springer Science+Business Media.

potential energy on release, the deceleration of the ball is a function of ball-pitch friction which is constant across the measured area. The measurement of green speed in golf using the Stimpmeter (USGA, 2009) is slightly different in that the ramp is raised manually by the operator – while this reduces the cost of equipment and increases the portability of the device, the control of release height is reduced and momentum can be imparted by the operator – affecting the ball roll distance.

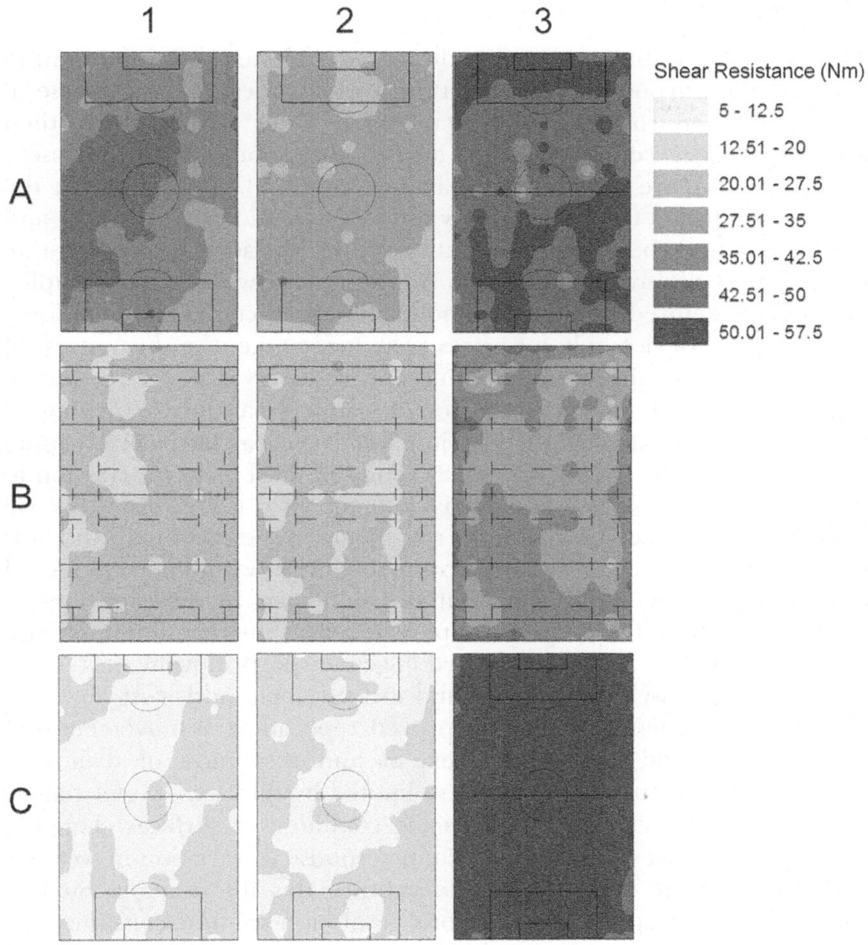


*Figure 8.6* Maps of shear resistance (traction/grip) measured with the GoingStick® from the three pitches (A, B, and C as per Figure 8.5) at three times across the season (1 = beginning of season; 2 = mid-season; 3 = end of season as per Figure 8.5). Reproduced from Caple et al. (2012), © International Sports Engineering Association, with kind permission of Springer Science+Business Media.

Ball rebound behaviour is more complex. Original methods looked at vertical ball rebound using a device that drops the ball normally onto the surface from a standard height, e.g. 3m for cricket and football (Mooney and Baker, 2000; Baker *et al.*, 2001) and measures the rebound height of the ball, which could then be compared to standard minimum and maximum rebound values or a range of coefficient of restitution. It is rare that the ball has a perfectly normal impact with the surface, so angled ball rebound behaviour is more representative but more difficult to achieve, commonly using air-cannon devices.

### *Development of improved devices*

To ensure that testing and testing devices are relevant, it is important to question the purpose of testing natural turf surfaces. If the purpose of testing is to improve the understanding of injury mechanisms, then improved, more complex testing devices that more closely represent human loading are required (see Chapters 4 and 7). This is because the rate of loading on the human body affects adaptation by the body, and the mechanical behaviour of natural turf surfaces is loading-rate dependent (Guisasola *et al.*, 2010b). An example of where more complex devices are required would be in understanding traction. The traditional studded-plate device only measures peak torque, i.e. the shear stress at failure and the strain rate is constant, and relatively slow (12 rev $min^{-1}$). Human loading of natural turf is more dynamic. In a study of turning on natural turf at a controlled speed of just 3.83m $s^{-1}$, peak horizontal loading rate was 2.98kN $s^{-1}$ (Guisasola, 2008). The soil must yield for traction to take place but the stress–strain behaviour for yield is critical as this will determine the rate of loading of the soft-tissues in the lower limb and how they accommodate this load. More complex devices would need to record force and deformation throughout the simulated turning movement, which would have to be more complex to reflect the magnitude of, and rotation of, stresses that are observed in actual sports movements.

Such complexity of movement and measurement adds cost however, so there is a trade-off between improved replication of movement and data capture, and the volume, extent and resolution of data sets. Epidemiological studies of injury are limited by the lack of explanatory surface characterisation data. With the condition of surfaces changing over short distances within the pitch in response to variation in weather and management, it is essential to capture this information. Surface surveys with high spatial and temporal resolution are time consuming so devices need to be rapid, portable and relatively low cost to encourage widespread adoption. This does not mean that data should be entirely irrelevant, more that it could be a simplification of the number of parameters measured, focusing on key information, or that it could be that peak values as opposed to whole force-displacement curves would be appropriate. An example would be in horseracing, where there is regular, systematic and obligatory testing of surfaces with devices such as the Going Stick providing valuable companion datasets for the epidemiology of racehorse injury (Williams *et al.*, 2001). These data do not explain injury mechanisms; they can only point to associations among injury rates, types of injury and surface parameters, but they do inform more detailed examination of horse–surface interaction and more complex simulation of loading in understanding injury mechanisms. There is a need for improved datasets in other sports such as football and rugby, both in terms of explaining injury mechanisms and in quantifying spatial and temporal variation in pitch performance that relate to injury incidence, especially as surface construction and management methods continue to evolve (Stiles *et al.*, 2009).

The current and future testing devices discussed here only quantify variation in performance parameters such as hardness and strength; they do not explain this variation. To manage spatial and temporal variation in natural turf sports surfaces requires detailed data on profile particle-size distribution, density, water content and organic matter content, requiring laboratory testing of samples of the soil offline. It is commonly variation in these parameters that is responsible for variation in pitch performance.

## Next-generation natural turf

It is common to discuss the development of synthetic turf in terms of 'generations' (see Chapter 2) – the first being short-pile nylon carpets, the second sand-filled 20–25mm polypropylene tufted fibres and the third sand- and rubber-filled longer-pile (40–65mm) tufted polypropylene/polyethylene fibre surfaces more suited to football and rugby. The transition from second- to third-generation synthetic turf is evolutionary (lengthening of fibres, inclusion of rubber infill) with the driver being improved replication of natural turf. Within a similar time frame, natural turf has been undergoing its own evolution in terms of construction (increase in sand profile pitches and hybrid surfaces) and management (increased irrigation and nutrient application, improved grass breeding and the use of supplementary growth lighting). The key difference is that this evolution has been restricted to elite-level stadium surfaces. Some advances in grass breeding and husbandry and also drainage construction have improved the quality of recreational surfaces but these remain cost-limited and therefore the benefits in performance from sand construction are not achievable. As part of the legacy of the London 2012 Olympics there has been government investment in the drainage and maintenance of natural turf surfaces through Sport England's Protecting Playing Fields scheme, which aims to improve the quality of natural turf sports surface provision to increase access to quality facilities and to improve participation.

Further development in natural turf technology is required in two key areas. The first is to increase wear resistance and carrying capacity of recreational surfaces. Solutions will need to be affordable and sustainable over the lifetime of a surface, which is commonly measured in decades at the recreational level. Surface performance is commonly limited by excess water in winter periods and insufficient water during summer periods. It follows that effective affordable drainage is essential but material selection and grass breeding must limit the effect of water shortage in dry periods, especially considering the projected effects of climate change. Developments in drainage technology must also consider the ongoing sustainability of funding, particularly where the effectiveness of drainage is dependent upon that funding, such as with sand-slitting for example.

The second is improved environmental sustainability of surface management. For natural turf surfaces to remain a competitive solution for sport in the future, when resource availability is expected to be reduced and population increased, it is essential to reduce the consumption of resources such as water, natural gas (used in the production of fertilisers), pesticides and minerals (James, 2011).

Elite-level surfaces could be engineered to improve performance and sustainability by providing real-time information on surface status. Within-surface sensor arrays could provide real-time information on turf stress and strength at a spatial resolution that reflects spatial variation in pitches. This would require the development of affordable, robust sensor technology for installation within a surface but would provide invaluable information for the improved management of surfaces, leading to reduced consumption and providing real-time and historical performance data. Current sensor technology is too expensive, too large and insufficiently robust for installation outside controlled research environments. Improved data recording could inform other aspects of surface management including the use of machinery. Bartlett and James (2011) showed how 21–54 per cent of the carbon footprint of golf course maintenance is from the use of mowing machinery. Machinery operation on golf courses is typically surface presentation optimised, which limits resource efficiency. Improved vehicle sensor technology is needed to inform optimisation of machinery operation in more resource-restricted environments.

If participation in sport increases in line with increase in population, then sports surfaces will need to provide greater carrying capacity for sport from a decreasing footprint as competition for space increases, particularly within urban environments. In parks and urban green space, then natural turf will continue to have a place in the urban environment as long as it can evolve to increase carrying capacity with reduced consumption. In schools and specialist sports facilities, synthetic turf will become more prevalent, because it has a greater carrying capacity. For sports such as golf and cricket, where large areas of turf are required and variation in surface conditions are desirable, then natural turf will remain the surface of choice at both recreational and elite level. The balance between natural and synthetic turf in the stadium environment for sports such as football is changing and the future will depend on the development of synthetic turf and whether it becomes more acceptable to elite participants, but also on the development of natural turf construction and management and whether its current playability and aesthetic advantages can be maintained sustainably.

## Key summary points

- Due principally to the low cost of construction, and to an extent historical factors, natural turf surfaces remain the most common and most extensive surfaces used for sport.
- The quality of a natural turf surface is directly proportional to the investment in construction, maintenance and resources and this can create a large divide between a small number of high-quality elite surfaces and a much larger number of lower-quality recreational surfaces where resources are much more constrained.
- Because natural turf systems are organic, they have a limited wear resistance but the potential for regeneration. This limits their sustainable usage compared to synthetic turf systems but with the right resource inputs they can provide the pinnacle of sports performance.
- Innovation, particularly in the construction and management of natural turf, has been accelerated in recent years by increasing demands from ever-improving player performance, increasing rewards for success and the demands of commercial broadcasters.
- Further development is needed at the recreational level to develop better performing, more sustainable natural turf surfaces that can complement the increasing provision of synthetic turf surfaces which can sustain a greater intensity of use per unit area.
- Sustainable development of natural turf has a key role to play in the provision of high-quality, accessible sports surfaces but access to maintenance expertise and resources is a key determinant in the quality of any natural turf surface.

## References

Baker, S. (1997) 'The reinforcement of turfgrass areas using plastic and other synthetic materials: A review', *International Turfgrass Society Research Journal*, 8: 3–13.

Baker, S. W., Hammond, L. K. and Stewart, K. F. (2001) 'Technical note: Influence of Clegg hammer weight on the relationship between surface hardness and ball rebound for cricket', *Journal of Turfgrass Science*, 76: 71–74.

Bartlett, M. D. and James, I. T. (2011) 'A model of greenhouse gas emissions from the management of turf on two golf courses', *Science of the Total Environment*, 409: 1357–1367.

BS EN 15301-1 (2007) *Surfaces for Sport Areas. Part 1: Determination of Rotational Resistance*. London: British Standards Institution.

Canaway, P. M. and Bell, M. J. (1986) 'Technical note: An apparatus measuring traction and friction on natural and artificial playing surfaces', *Journal of the Sports Turf Research Institute*, 62: 211–214.

Caple, M., James, I. and Bartlett, M. (2012) 'Spatial analysis of the mechanical behaviour of natural turf sports pitches', *Sports Engineering*, 15: 143–157.

Chivers, I. and Aldous, D. (2004) 'Performance monitoring of grassed playing surfaces for Australian rules football', *Journal of Turfgrass and Sports Surface Science*, 70: 73–80.

Dufour, M.J.D. and Mumford, C. (2008) 'GoingStick® technology and electromagnetic induction scanning for naturally-turfed sports surfaces', *Sports Technology*, 1: 125–131.

Guisasola, I. N. (2008) 'Human – natural sports surface interaction', unpublished thesis, Cranfield University, UK. Online. Available at: http://hdl.handle.net/1826/3487 (accessed 31 January 2011).

Guisasola, I., James, I., Llewellyn, C., Stiles, V. and Dixon, S. (2010a) 'Quasi-static mechanical behaviour of soils used for natural turf sports surfaces and stud force prediction', *Sports Engineering*, 12: 99–109.

Guisasola, I., James, I. Stiles, V. and Dixon, S. (2010b) 'Dynamic behaviour of soils used for natural turf sports surfaces', *Sports Engineering*, 12: 111–122.

ISO 11277 (2009) *Soil quality – Determination of Particle Size Distribution in Mineral Soil Material – Method by Sieving and Sedimentation*. Geneva: International Organization for Standardization.

James, I. T. (2011) 'Advancing natural turf to meet tomorrow's challenges', *Proceedings of the Institution of Mechanical Engineers Part P: Journal of Sports Engineering and Technology*, 225: 115–129.

James, I. T., Blackburn, D.W.K. and Godwin, R. J. (2007) 'Mole drainage as an alternative to sand slitting in natural turf sports surfaces on clays', *Soil Use and Management*, 23: 28–35.

McNitt, A. S. and Landschoot, P. J. (2005) 'The effects of soil reinforcing materials on the traction and divot resistance of a sand root zone', *International Turfgrass Society Research Journal*, 10: 1115–1122.

Mooney, S. J. and Baker, S. W. (2000) 'The effects of grass cutting height and pre-match rolling and watering on football pitch ground cover and playing quality', *Journal of Turfgrass Science*, 76: 70–77.

Sport England (2011) *Natural Turf for Sport Design Guidance Note*. London: Sport England. Online. Available at: www.sportengland.org/media/30865/Natural-turf-for-sport.pdf

Stiles, V. H., James, I. T., Dixon, S. J. and Guisasola, I. N. (2009) 'Natural turf surfaces: The case for continued research', *Sports Medicine*, 39: 65–84.

Twomey, D. (2010) 'Is there a link between injury and ground conditions? A case study in Australian Football', Presented at the 2nd Science Technology and Research in Sports Surfaces (STARSS II) Conference, Loughborough, UK, 21–22 April.

USGA (2009) *Stimpmeter Instruction Booklet*, Far Hills, NJ: United States Golf Association. Online. Available at: www.usga.org/course_care/articles/management/greens/Stimpmeter-Instruction-Booklet/ (accessed 28 January 2011).

Ward, C. J. (1983) 'Sports turf drainage: A review', *Journal of the Sports Turf Research Institute*, 59: 9–28.

Williams, R. B., Harkin, L. S., Hammond, C. J. and Wood, J.L.N. (2001) 'Predominance of tendon injuries on British racecourses (flat racing and national hunt racing)', in R. B. Williams, E. Houghton and J. F. Wade (eds) *Proceedings of the 13th International Conference of Racing Analysts and Veterinarians*. Newmarket, UK: R and W Publications, pp. 274–277.

Chapter 9

# The future of sports surfaces

*Sharon Dixon, Paul Fleming, Iain James and Matt Carré*

## Introduction

This chapter considers possible directions regarding the future development of sports surfaces, drawing on the areas highlighted in each of the preceding chapters. This includes: future directions in natural turf and synthetic surface construction; development of refined mechanical test methods; improved understanding of the mechanical interaction between footwear and surface; and greater understanding of human interaction in terms of injury risk and performance. The potential social impacts of surface developments are also considered.

## Future challenges in sports surface construction – natural turf and synthetic surfaces

In Chapter 2, the challenge to provide sports facilities in terms of the growing population and increased urbanisation was highlighted. This was linked with an increased demand to provide sports surfaces that are weather and wear resistant, with a focus on the need to consider the impact of water on the performance and durability of the surface. This challenge exists for both synthetic and natural turf surfaces. Modern sports complexes include a combination of natural turf and synthetic turf surfaces that allow the synthetic turf surfaces to be used for training and community use with natural turf stadium pitches for elite-level performance. This mixed model allows sports facilities to be delivered on a smaller footprint. The trend towards increasing installation of synthetic turf will continue – driven by economics. The trade-off between performance and durability has to be overcome. Continued materials development is required to maximise life cycle, minimise injury risk and maximise carrying capacity, while maintaining acceptable performance. The impact of sports surface development on resource consumption and environmental impacts such as flooding must be considered in future sports surface design. This will include a reduction in water and fossil fuel use in production and maintenance and more sustainable design to attenuate water to prevent off-site flooding. This inevitably requires advances in both above-ground and below-ground engineering.

An increased trend to develop multi-use facilities was also described in Chapter 2. Since most sports have specific requirements in terms of player and ball interaction, there is a key design challenge in terms of the development of surfaces that achieve required performance standards for a range of sports. This is while also coping with the additional usage associated with a community-based multi-use synthetic surface. We have seen changes in some sports as a result of play on synthetic surfaces, most notably in field hockey (as described in Chapter 2). The increased use of multi-sports surfaces in elite and community sports is likely to see further adaptation across a range of sports in the future. The requirements of the surfaces themselves may also change in the future due to trends in usage, such as the increased popularity of five-/six-a-side football recreation centres, which have increased hours of play per week compared to more traditional eleven-a-side school/amateur club football pitches.

As well as the requirements of the local community influencing sports surface construction, the provision of a common surface for a range of sports is increasingly influencing the culture of individual sports and thus having a social impact. For example, Saturday morning youth football in the UK is increasingly making use of artificial surfaces to provide a playing surface across the entire weekend. The availability of these surfaces for repeated use without a requirement for recovery (as for natural turf) reduces the number of postponed games, but has a social impact in terms of when the game is played and the structure of the family weekend. Similarly, training for a range of sports can now take place late into the evening, making good use of the available facilities but again having a social impact. We increasingly see a requirement for flexibility in many aspects of life, and a flexible approach to the scheduling of sports participation appears to also be part of this evolution, influenced by significant developments in sports surface design and technology. The mixed-surface facility can therefore provide a range of options for use.

Another important consideration is the distance players and families are willing to travel to participate in sport. This is a key factor when investing in community sport facilities and there is a limit to the cost and time that can be spent before participation declines. Therefore it is important to have access to good facilities locally. A full-sized third-generation (3G) football pitch could cost at least £600,000. The cost of draining and improving a natural turf football pitch would be approximately £60,000. It follows that for every synthetic turf pitch, ten existing natural turf pitches could be improved. In terms of usage, particularly during the winter, the 3G pitch could be used more than the ten natural turf pitches together at a much lower maintenance cost, but the geographical spread of facilities would be much lower, with people living in smaller, more rural communities having to travel much further to access sports facilities. This is why a mixed model of facility provision is required.

## Future development and application of mechanical test methods

A clear challenge identified in Chapters 3, 6 and 7 is the development of mechanical test methods that adequately simulate human–surface interaction and reproduce sport-specific shoe–surface combinations. The increasing focus on the surface role in sporting performance and safety/injury risk demands more biofidelic evaluation testing. In terms of simulating human interaction with the surface, Chapter 3 highlighted the current compromise in providing tests that are relatively simple (often pseudo-static for example), portable and repeatable, and thus are not simulative of player loading. Advances require the application of more relevant high rates of dynamic loading in more than one direction simultaneously, to better simulate the surface demands during real sports movements. Some novel devices have been developed, but have remained largely as research prototypes. However, there is likely to remain a need for simple portable tests that provide useful comparison between surfaces and monitor changes over time.

A key question to consider is why the surface is being quantified mechanically. One reason is for standardisation, to ensure all surfaces provided for a particular application have consistent characteristics. This approach ensures that surfaces for certain sports have reliable characteristics, although only for the specific characteristics that the test method quantifies (i.e. force reduction when impacted with a defined impact energy). There are many simple, mechanical test devices that are suitably reliable that could be used to ensure repeatability of defined surface characteristics. However, with much evidence that ranking of surfaces is highly sensitive to the specific impact conditions (see Chapters 3 and 7), it seems that quantifying a surface property such as hardness with a single test method is likely to be misleading. This approach tells us very little, if anything, about the ability of the surface to permit optimum performance with minimal injury risk. Of more concern, it is possible that providing the optimum performance and safety of surfaces (in real-world loading conditions) could be hampered by the current tests and standards.

An alternative approach is to utilise mechanical test devices to assess whether a surface is safe for participation and/or appropriate in terms of performance. For example, if it were known that surfaces providing mechanical cushioning within certain defined limits (measured by a specific device) were safer in terms of injury risk than surfaces with properties outside of these limits, then this device has a clear application. While this seems to be the aim of some of the governing bodies when specifying the use of mechanical test devices, there is a lack of solid evidence relating mechanical test data to injury risk or performance. Some advances have been made, for example as described in Chapter 4, but more evidence of relationships between mechanical test results and injury and performance is required to confidently take this approach with existing mechanical test devices. An 'ideal' multidisciplinary research-led approach is described in more detail at the end of this chapter.

The application of mechanical test devices to provide a detailed characterisation of sports surface behaviour, as opposed to pass/fail evaluation, is suggested as an alternative focus for mechanical test devices. For example, a thorough mechanical characterisation of a surface to provide measures such as hardness, stiffness and damping, over a range of loading conditions, can be used to provide a unique description of the surface of interest. Knowledge of biomechanical human response to changes in each of these parameters would be a first step to understanding the effect of surface properties on human behaviour. Once surface characterisation is established and resultant biomechanical responses are documented, relationships with injury patterns or performance on the surface could be explored. Thus, as well as a focus being required on the development of tests to adequately simulate conditions of human–surface interaction during sports participation (as indicated in Chapter 3), it is suggested that one avenue for future work is to characterise surfaces more fully and to perform systematic study of the influence of defined surface characteristics on human biomechanics.

## Future approaches to improving understanding of shoe–surface interaction

As described in Chapter 6, an understanding of shoe–surface interaction is dependent on the development of appropriate mechanical test methods. A requirement for obtaining biomechanical measurements during 'in-game' situations is suggested in Chapter 3, providing data on the loads applied to sports surfaces and thus informing the development of appropriate test methods for understanding shoe–surface interaction.

The obtaining of biomechanical data during actual sports participation should be facilitated by recent developments in force and movement sensor technology. Increasingly motion capture systems, such as those described in Chapter 7, can provide suitably accurate and reliable data when used in an outside environment. This increasingly permits the collection of good kinematic data in a sporting environment. In addition, developments in wireless sensor technology increasingly permit the measurement of movement and force in a competitive sports environment with minimal interference with the athlete (Cheung *et al.*, 2010). Advances in miniaturisation of sensors has permitted the quantification of shear load, for example in individual soccer cleats (Matsuo *et al.*, 2011). Improvements in affordability also mean that it may soon be routine to measure shear forces experienced by the outside of shoe soles.

All of these advances can provide detailed data on the requirements of a mechanical test device to apply loads to investigate shoe–surface interaction in a controlled manner. The Sheffield device described in Chapter 6 makes use of biomechanical data that were collected specifically to obtain boundary conditions for the loads during shoe–surface interaction for typical tennis movements. However, the biomechanical data collected to inform the development of this device were obtained within a laboratory environment, limiting the ecological validity of the data. This approach was used because of limitations in both the motion analysis (kinematic) and force plate data collection systems – controlled lighting conditions were required for the motion analysis system and a suitable force plate mounting was required. Recent developments in both the areas of motion analysis and force data collection, as described earlier in this section, are increasing the ability to collect data in true sporting environments. This enhances the quality and suitability of biomechanical data used to develop mechanical test devices, and thus improves our ability to understand factors influencing shoe–surface interaction. By interrogating the results obtained from mechanical test devices and examining the tribological mechanisms that occur (as discussed in Chapter 6), deeper understanding can be provided to ensure that the relevant physics of the problem is replicated. This can also inform future modelling approaches and the creation of portable devices.

## Relating human–surface interaction to injury risk and performance optimisation

Chapter 4 highlighted the need for collection of biomechanical and injury data for defined surface conditions, so that specific biomechanical responses can be related to injury risk. One suggested approach for integrated study design is illustrated in Figure 9.1. This model involves the identification of surfaces with differing characteristics that are utilised in sports activities, monitoring play on these surfaces for different populations (sports teams, running clubs etc.), and characterising each of the surfaces mechanically. Specific mechanical characteristics, such as cushioning behaviour, will therefore be known, alongside the frequency of play on each surface. Biomechanical data collection should be performed for the populations performing on the surfaces, thus revealing any biomechanical differences, such as different movement patterns and

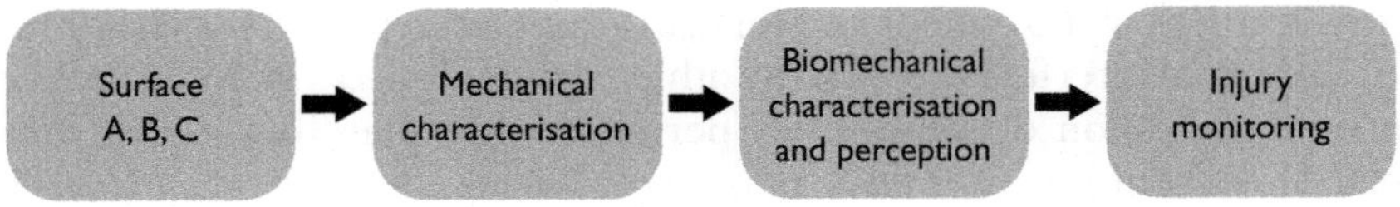


*Figure 9.1* Suggested process for improving understanding of biomechanical mechanisms for surface-related injury.

loading under the foot. At the same time as monitoring frequency of surface use, injury monitoring should take place for each of the study populations. At the end of the study period, associations between surface type (mechanical characteristics) and biomechanics and injury should be investigated, revealing specific biomechanical mechanisms for injury on the surfaces.

As highlighted in Chapter 5, while there is reasonable understanding of some of the biomechanical responses to a change in surface, most studies do not consider in sufficient depth the influence of these changes on human performance. However, Chapter 5 also describes the emergence of laboratory-based studies of sports surfaces and biomechanics which do include some measure of performance. For example, time taken to execute typical sports movements such as sprints and agility courses has been recorded for different shoe–surface traction (see Chapter 5). These results have then been related to the biomechanical measure of utilised traction. A subsequent study also quantified joint moments for the studied shoe–surface combinations (Schrier *et al.*, 2014). A greater number of studies which include measures of performance and biomechanics should improve our understanding of relationships between these measures, informing the development of surfaces to optimise performance and minimise injury risk.

## The importance of multidisciplinary studies

Engineering studies to identify materials and constructions that provide defined mechanical characteristics are important for the development of reliable, durable and sustainable sports surfaces. Engineering approaches to the understanding of shoe–surface interaction in terms of mechanical test devices and materials modelling are also important. Of equal importance is the performance of biomechanical studies for different surfaces to improve understanding of human response to defined surface characteristics, and to relate this to injury and performance. However, we suggest that multidisciplinary studies which combine mechanical characterisation, quantification of human behaviour and perception, shoe–surface and human modelling, and monitoring of injury and performance, are required to fully understand the influence of the sports surface on the performer and thus to optimise surface design. An increasing number of studies are adopting the suggested integrated approach described in Chapter 4, quantifying both mechanical and biomechanical behaviour (Zanetti *et al.*, 2014; Carré *et al.*, 2014). The addition of player perception measures (e.g. Fleming *et al.*, 2005) and physiological variables such as heart rate and energy cost (Brito *et al.*, 2012) will further develop our understanding of surfaces. There are already examples of modelling of the surface or shoe–surface combination (e.g. Baroud *et al.*, 1999; Davidson *et al.*, 2009) and models of human interaction with surfaces (e.g. Maquirriain, 2013). The performance of multidisciplinary studies will further progress our understanding of injury and performance effects and our ability to develop more relevant mechanical test methods. This combined approach will also inform the development of player–shoe–surface models and thus our ability to develop optimal surface designs, as illustrated in Figure 9.2.

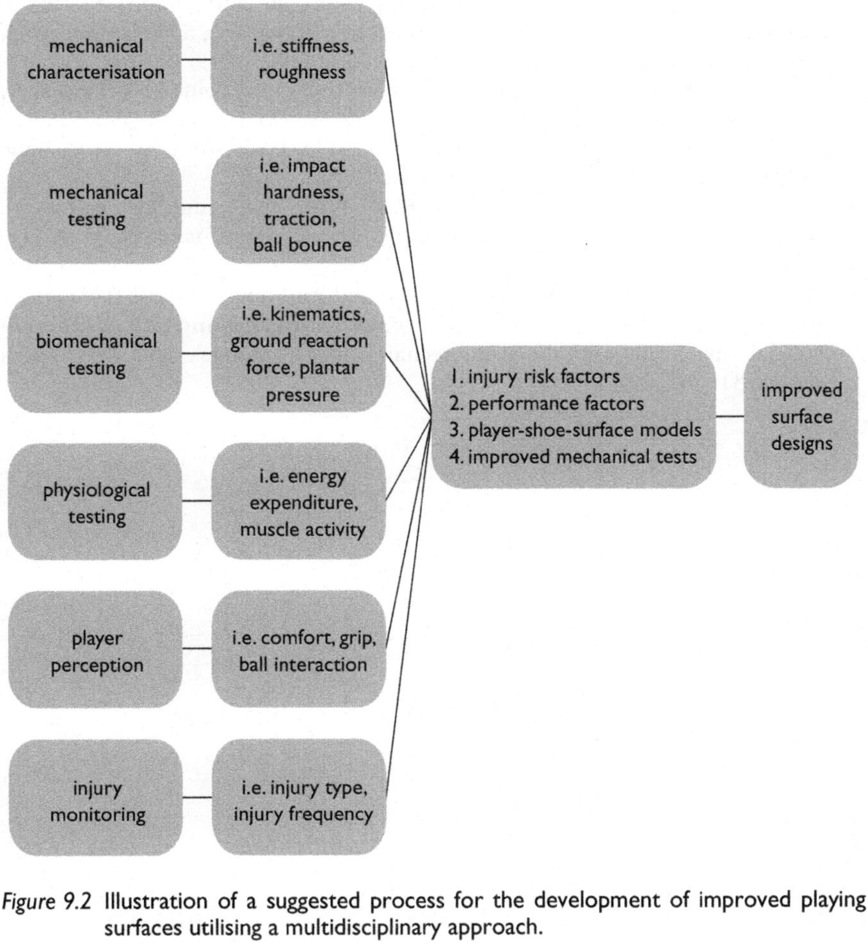


*Figure 9.2* Illustration of a suggested process for the development of improved playing surfaces utilising a multidisciplinary approach.

## References


Baroud, G., Nigg, B. M. and Stefanyshyn, D. (1999) 'Energy storage and return in sport surfaces', *Sports Engineering,* 2: 173–180.

Brito, J., Krustrup, P. and Rebelo, A. (2012) 'The influence of the playing surface on the exercise intensity of small-sided recreational soccer games', *Human Movement Science,* 31: 946–956.

Carré, M., Clarke, J., Damm, L. and Dixon, S. (2014) 'Friction at the tennis shoe–court interface: how biomechanically informed lab-based testing can enhance understanding', *Procedia Engineering*, 72: 883–888.

Cheung, L., Tan, H., Kuntze, K., Lowe, J., Bezodis, I. N., Hailes, S., Wilson, A. and Kerwin, D. (2010) 'Sensing for stride information of sprinters', *Wireless Sensor Networks, Lecture Notes in Computer Science*, 5970: 147–161.

Davidson, P. L., Wilson, S. J., Wilson, B. D. and Chalmers, D. J. (2009) 'An approach to modeling impact energy absorption by surfaces', *Journal of Applied Biomechanics*, 25: 351–359.

Fleming, P. R., Young, C., Roberts, J. R., Jones, R. and Dixon, N. (2005) 'Human perceptions of artificial surfaces for field hockey', *Sports Engineering*, 8: 121–136, ISEA.

Maquirriain, J. (2013) 'The interaction between the tennis court and the player: How does surface affect leg stiffness?', *Sports Biomechanics*, 12: 48–53.

Matsuo, K., Moriyasu, K. and Nishiwaki, T. (2011) 'Basic study on cleat shape design in soccer boots', *Footwear Science*, 3, S1: S101–102.

Schrier, N. M., Wannop, J. W., Lewinson, R. T., Worobets, J. and Stefanyshyn, D. (2014) 'Shoe traction and surface compliance affect performance of soccer-related movements', *Footwear Science*, 6: 69–80.

Zanetti, E. M., Bignardi, C., Franceschini, G. and Audenino, A. (2014) 'Amateur football pitches: Mechanical properties of the natural ground and of different artificial turf infills and their biomechanical implications', *Journal of Sports Sciences*, 31: 767–778.

# Glossary

## Physics/engineering terms

**Coefficient of friction** Ratio of friction force to normal force between two interacting bodies such as the shoe and surface.

**Coefficient of restitution** The ratio of rebound velocity to impact velocity. This term is often used to express energy recovery of a ball to surface impact.

**Compliance** The corollary to stiffness and deformation, a compliant surface is 'relatively' easy to deform.

**Damping** Resistance to motion under dynamic loading, related to the velocity of motion. As damping increases peak deformation decreases.

**Deflection/deformation** The movement of a surface under an applied load, usually refers to a dynamic load. Direction should be specified, e.g. vertical. Can be elastic or plastic.

**Displacement** The movement of a surface under an applied load, usually refers to a static load. Direction should be specified. Can be elastic or plastic.

**Elastic stiffness** The ratio of applied force to recoverable deflection (e.g. in a linear spring).

**Form-locking** Penetration of surface by footwear.

**Friction** The resistance to relative motion of two planar surfaces in contact. Can be expressed as static (initial movement) or dynamic (constant velocity) friction and be due to different mechanisms (e.g. adhesion, hysteresis).

**Grip or traction** Grip is often expressed colloquially as the underfoot friction developed between the shoe and surface (often used for indoor floors and tennis). In many cases the shoe or surface are non-planar, such that grip can be defined as the resistance to relative motion of two non-planar surfaces in contact. However, traction is the term often used to express the resistance of a studded boot to a compliant surface (such as natural turf and artificial grass). These terms can be expressed as static or dynamic grip or traction. They can also be measured due to a rotational or translational (straight-line) movement.

**Hardness** Resistance to penetration (e.g. shore hardness of rubber). Often used to mean shock absorbency, resistance to deformation.

**Hysteresis** An expression for energy loss for a material during cycle(s) of loading/unloading due to some plasticity behaviour in elastic materials.

**Impact attenuation** Dissipation of the kinetic energy of an impact by localised deformation or displacement such that the (peak) acceleration is reduced.

**Material strength** The stress applied to cause rupture (can be tensile, shear etc.).

**Roughness** A measurement of the topographical profile of a surface, often to the order of microns.

**Shear strength (soil)** The ultimate limit (peak) of shear stress applied to cause a plastic failure surface to develop.

**Shock-absorbency** The measurable ability for a surface to reduce the peak force under a controlled or uncontrolled impact.

**Stiffness** The ratio of force to deflection.

**Torque** Product of the magnitude of force and the perpendicular distance from the line of action of the force to the axis of rotation.

**Tribology** Study of interacting surfaces in relative motion.

**Viscoelastic** Exhibiting both viscous and elastic behaviour when deformed, resulting in combined damping and stiffness.

## Natural turf terms

**Aerobic** Requiring the presence of air (oxygen), for example processes such as respiration in plants and humans.

**Anoxic** The complete absence of oxygen, for example in a soil.

**(Apparent) Cohesion** Cohesion is the intermolecular bonding of a substance. Clay soils exhibit this property as inter-molecular forces between individual *phyllosilicate* clay minerals form a vital component of soil strength. Apparent cohesion is more apparent in sandy soils dominated by silica minerals. The strength in sandy soils comes from inter-particle friction between individual grains and aggregates of grains. The strength of a sand soil can increase with addition of small quantities of water which adhere to the sand particles creating an apparent cohesion similar to that of true cohesion among clay minerals. Increasing water content further decreases apparent cohesion as the distance between sand particles increases and friction is reduced.

**Capillary action** The process whereby a fluid such as water can flow in a narrow tube or pore due to the balance between internal (within the liquid) cohesive forces and external (between the liquid and the tube/pore wall) adhesive forces. Capillary action is a component of water movement in soils and plants.

**Compaction** The increase in bulk density of a soil under load, typically from the surface, such as foot or vehicle traffic, the use of rollers or temporary structures. The consequence of compaction is usually a reduction in *hydraulic conductivity* and infiltration rate and rate of gas movement and exchange in the soil. These result in poorer conditions for grass growth (undesirable) and an increase in both hardness and stiffness which can affect both player–surface and ball–surface interactions.

**Hydraulic conductivity** A property of soils and plants that describes the ease of movement of water through a soil (see Darcy's Law). Water movement is predominantly in the pore network between solid particles. Hydraulic conductivity is inversely proportional to pore size and therefore decreases with decreasing particle size and as dry bulk density is increased through *compaction*.

**Photosynthesis** Grass plants convert light energy, carbon dioxide and water into chemical energy stored as carbohydrates that are used in other metabolic processes that drive grass growth and development. This occurs in the two-stage process of photosynthesis. Briefly, in the first light-dependent stage, light energy, water and carbon dioxide are converted in specialist cells to produce oxygen, electrons for biochemical reactions and two important compounds, nicotinamide adenine dinucleotide phosphate (NADPH) and adenosine triphosphate (ATP). These compounds are used in the second, light-independent, stage to produce sugars and other carbohydrates in the Krebs cycle.

**Phyllosilicate** Clay minerals are alumina phyllosilicates which are sheet-forming minerals in the Earth's crust, and are typically weathering products from other minerals such as feldspar. These minerals comprise sheets of $SiO_4$ tetrahedra and $AlO_4$ octahedra. The combination of sheets results in a net-negative surface charge on the mineral lattice that requires a balancing cation such as calcium or magnesium which can then become hydrated, causing the mineral to expand on wetting.

**Plastic** Most deformation in soils is plastic, unrecoverable deformation and dependent upon the stress path.

**Respiration** Respiration is the metabolism of sugars (formed by *photosynthesis*) within the plant in the presence of oxygen to produce energy, carbon dioxide and water. Turfgrass plant roots will respire within the soil, requiring oxygen and emitting carbon dioxide. Aeration is a key process in turf management that allows oxygen to reach plant roots from the atmosphere and carbon dioxide concentrations to be reduced before they become toxic.

**Silica** Silicon-dioxide $SiO_2$, which in its natural mineral form is quartz. Quartz is a highly abundant mineral on Earth and forms the majority of sand particles in soils.

**Transpiration** In turfgrasses, water enters the plant roots through osmosis and moves upwards under capillary action and gradients in hydraulic potential towards the stomata (microscopic holes) in the plant leaves. This process, in which the plant is active, is known as transpiration and results in the transport of water, hormones, soluble nutrients and salts around the plant, and provides *turgor* to keep the plant upright.

**Turgor** Turgor pressure within plant cells, provides rigidity at the cellular and whole plant level. The turgidity is driven by osmosis as water moves into cells under a solute gradient. Thus without water and the correct nutrients, plants will lose turgidity and rigidity and be more susceptible to damage from wear. The change in rigidity also affects ball-surface interactions in sports such as golf and tennis.

## Biomechanical terms

**Abduction** Movement of a segment away from the midline.

**Acute injury** Injury as a result of a single event.

**Adduction** Movement of a segment towards the midline.

**Anterior** Positioned in front of a defined reference point.

**Available friction/traction** Maximum friction/traction that exists to affect player movements, resulting from the properties of the shoe and surface.

**Bursa** A fibrous fluid-filled sac typically between bones and tendons, reducing friction during movement.

**Bursitis** Inflammation of the bursa.

**Centre of gravity** Point about which gravitational force is balanced. Typically coincides with centre of mass.

**Centre of mass** Point about which the mass is distributed equally.

**Chronic injury** Injury that develops over time as a result of repeated, continuous load on a structure.

**Dorsi-flexion** Rotation of the foot towards the shin in the sagittal plane.

**Electromyography** Measurement of the electrical activity of a muscle.

**Epidemiological studies** Investigation of the patterns and causes of injury or illness in defined populations.

**Eversion** Rotation of the foot in the frontal plane such that the lateral border of the foot is lifted and the foot sole moves to face away from the midline of the body.

**Extension** Movement of a segment away from an adjacent segment so that the angle between segments is increased.

**Flexion** Movement of a segment towards an adjacent segment so that the angle between segments is reduced.

**Force platform** Device used to measure dynamic ground reaction forces.

**Frontal plane** Plane that bisects the body into front and back halves.

**Ground reaction force** Resultant force as a result of contact between a human and the ground, typically measured with a force platform.

**Hallux** Big toe.

**Hamstrings** Group of muscles on the back of the thigh.

**Hyperextension** Extension of a joint beyond the neutral orientation.

**Impact peak** High frequency peak that occurs when two objects collide – used to describe the impact force occurring within the first 50 ms of foot–ground contact during heel–toe running.

**Internal knee abductor moment (knee external adductor moment)** Moment that tends to abduct the knee.

**Internal knee adductor moment (knee external abductor moment)** Moment that tends to adduct the knee.

**Inverse dynamics** Estimation of internal forces and moments using external force, kinematic and segmental inertia data.

**Inversion** Rotation of the foot in the frontal plane such that the medial side of the foot is lifted and the foot sole moves to face the midline of the body.

**Joint moment** Net rotational effect of forces acting about a joint.

**Kinematics** Study of spatial and temporal components of motion.

**Kinetics** Study of the forces acting on a system.

**Knee abduction** Movement of the knee towards the midline of the body (medially).

**Knee adduction** Movement of the knee away from the midline of the body (laterally).

**Lateral** Positioned relatively further from the midline of the body.

**Ligament** Fibrous cord connecting two bones.

**Medial** Positioned relatively closer to the midline of the body.

**Medial tibial stress syndrome** Pain of the medial side of the lower leg, as a result of repeated trauma of the connective tissue surrounding the tibia. Also referred to as 'shin splints'.

**Minimal shoes** Footwear designed to simulate barefoot running, with negligible cushioning or structural support.

**Osteoarthritis** Degenerative disease of the joint, involving degradation of articular cartilage and subchondral bone.

**Plantar fascia** Fibrous band running along the plantar surface of the foot.

**Plantar fasciitis** Inflammation of the plantar fascia.

**Plantar-flexion** Rotation of the foot away from the shin in the sagittal plane (pointing the toes).

**Plantar pressure** Pressure beneath the foot.Posterior: Positioned behind a defined reference point.

**Potential energy** Energy stored in an object as a result of its position.

**Pressure** Force divided by contact area.

**Pronation** Combined abduction, eversion and dorsiflexion of the foot in relation to the lower leg.

**Prospective study** A study that monitors a defined outcome (such as injury) in a group of subjects over time, and relates this to defined risk or protection factors.

**Quadriceps** Group of muscles on the front of the thigh.

**Retrospective study** A study that looks backwards over time to quantify exposure to defined risk or protection factors in relation to a defined outcome (such as injury).

**Sagittal Plane** Plane that bisects the body into left and right sides.

**Tendinopathy** Inflammation of the tendon ('tendinitis') and/or microtears in the connective tissue in or around the tendon ('tendinosis').

**Tendon** Fibrous cord connecting muscle to bone.

**Torsion** Frontal plane rotation of the forefoot relative to the rearfoot.

**Transverse plane** Plane that is perpendicular to the long axis of the body.

**Utilised traction** Amount of traction that the performer uses during a specific movement.

**Valgus** Segment angle inclined medially.

**Varus** Segment angle inclined laterally.

## Artificial Surface Terms

**Approved turf product** A specified and unique combination of carpet and shock pad which has been tested by an FIH-accredited laboratory and verified as meeting the requirements in this handbook and the conditions laid down in the licensing agreement.

**Carpet** The topmost layer of woven, tufted or knitted materials of a turf.

**Certified pitch** A pitch which has been tested by an FIH-accredited laboratory and verified as meeting the requirements in this handbook and the conditions laid down in the licensing agreement. The pitch carpet must be the carpet from an approved product but the shock pad may be as specified for that approved product or may be a pre-existing shock pad. If it is a pre-existing shock pad, it must be from another product which was an approved product at the time of installation of the shock pad.

**Class I certificate** The certificate issued to a pitch which meets the full (class 1) set of field test requirements in this handbook.

**Class 2 certificate** The certificate issued to a pitch which meets the limited (class 2) set of field test requirements in this handbook.

**Global turf** A synthetic turf supplied by a licensed manufacturer which has been shown by independent laboratory testing by an FIH-accredited laboratory to meet the (top) global level performance requirements in this handbook.

**Licensing agreement** The formal agreement entered into by a turf manufacturer and the FIH governing the conditions under which approval of turf products may be granted.

**Licensed manufacturer** A synthetic turf manufacturer who has entered a licensing agreement with FIH. In this handbook and in the licensing agreement, 'manufacturer' also includes a supplier who has entered a licensing agreement with FIH, but who is not necessarily itself a manufacturer.

**National turf** A synthetic turf supplied by a licensed manufacturer which has been shown by independent laboratory testing by an FIH-accredited laboratory to meet the national level performance requirements in this handbook.

**Permeability** Capacity of a turf or pitch to transmit water by infiltration, drainage and absorption of the water through the carpet and shock pad to the structure immediately below.

**Pile** The full depth of tufts or loops of yarn which form the carpet.

**Shock pad** Resilient material under the pitch carpet to absorb kinetic energy. Sometimes referred to as 'shock absorbing layer', 'elastic layer' or 'e-layer'.

**Sub-base** The engineered support structure for a synthetic pitch.

**Yarn** Material used for tufts or loops to manufacture the carpet.

# Index